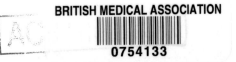
The Royal College of Anaesthetists has removed ~~... ...~~ ...ng from all MCQ examinations with effect from September 2008.

The version of the QBase Interactive Examination software on the CD-ROM that accompanies this volume is QBase Plus for non-negatively marked examinations. Correct answers receive one mark. There is no penalty for an incorrect answer or for a question left unanswered. Candidates should answer all the questions.

Installation instructions

Insert the **QBase CD** into the CD drive of your computer.

Double click the **Setup.exe** icon on the CD and follow the onscreen instructions.

Select the **Typical** Installation Option and accept the default directory for installation of QBase Plus.

The installation program will create a folder called **QBase Plus** on your hard disk and in the Start Menu.

To Run QBase Plus, either double click the **QBase Plus** icon in the QBase Plus folder or select **QBase Plus.exe** from the Start Menue by going to Start>Programs>QBase Plus>QBase Plus.exe.

The questions on any QBase CD work with either the original version of QBase or QBase Plus. Once you have installed the QBase Plus software, you can use any of the Anaesthesia CDs. Remember that, for non-negative marking exams, you should select the QBase Plus program and not QBase after you have inserted the CD into the drive.

Ed Hammond and Andrew McIndoe
QBase editors
June 2008

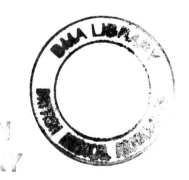

QBASE ANAESTHESIA 5
MCQs FOR THE FINAL FRCA

QBASE ANAESTHESIA 5
MCQs FOR THE FINAL FRCA

Karine Zander
Julius Cranshaw
John Isaac
Sundeep Karadia
David Lockey
Judith Nolan
Andrew Padkin
Richard Protheroe
Jonathan Williams

Edited by
Edward Hammond MA, BM BCh, MRCP, FRCA
Consultant Anaesthetist
Royal Devon & Exeter Hospital

Andrew K, McIndoe MB ChB, FRCA
Consultant Anaesthetist
Sir Humphry Davy Department of Anaesthesia
Bristol Royal Infirmary

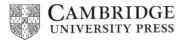
CAMBRIDGE
UNIVERSITY PRESS

CAMBRIDGE
UNIVERSITY PRESS

University Printing House, Cambridge CB2 8BS, United Kingdom

Published in the United States of America by Cambridge University Press, New York

Cambridge University Press is part of the University of Cambridge.

It furthers the University's mission by disseminating knowledge in the pursuit of education, learning and research at the highest international levels of excellence.

www.cambridge.org
Information on this title: www.cambridge.org/97805210521677059

© Cambridge University Press 2005

First published 2005
7th printing 2017

Printed in the United Kingdom by Print on Demand, World Wide

A catalogue record for this publication is available from the British Library

ISBN-13: 978-0-521-67705-9 Paperback

Every effort has been made in preparing this publication to provide accurate and up-to-date information which is in accord with accepted standards and practice at the time of publication. Although case histories are drawn from actual cases, every effort has been made to disguise the identities of the individuals involved. Nevertheless, the authors, editors and publishers can make no warranties that the information contained herein is totally free from error, not least because clinical standards are constantly changing through research and regulation. The authors, editors and publishers therefore disclaim all liability for direct or consequential damages resulting from the use of material contained in this publication. Readers are strongly advised to pay careful attention to information provided by the manufacturer of any drugs or equipment that they plan to use.

Contents

Installation Instructions

MINIMUM SYSTEM REQUIREMENTS

- An IBM compatible PC with a 80386 processor and 4 MB of RAM
- VGA monitor set up to display at least 256 colours
- CD-ROM drive
- Windows 95 or higher with Microsoft compatible mouse

NB: The display setting of your computer must be set to display 'SMALL FONTS' (see MS Windows manuals for further instructions on how to do this if necessary)

INSTALLATION INSTRUCTIONS

The program will install the appropriate files onto your hard drive. It requires the QBase CD-ROM to be in installed in the CD-ROM drive (usually drives D: or E:)

In order to run QBase, the CD must be in the drive

Print **Readme.txt** and **Helpfile.txt** on the CD-ROM for fuller instructions and user manual

WINDOWS 95, 98, 2000, XP

1. Insert the QBase CD-ROM into the drive
2. From the Start Menu, select the Run... option, type **D:\setup.exe** (where D: is the CD-ROM drive) and press OK or **OR** open the contents of the CD-ROM and double-click the **setup.exe** icon
3. Follow the 'Full – install all files' to accept the default directory for installation of QBase
4. Click 'Yes' to the prompt 'Do you want setup to create Program Manager groups?' If you have a previously installed version of QBase, click 'Yes' to the next prompt 'Should the new Program Manager groups replace existing duplicate groups?'

To run QBase, go to the Start Menu, then Programs, QBase and **QBase Exam**. From Windows Explorer, double-click the **QBase.exe** file in the QBase folder on your hard drive.

Editor's Note

The examination

The Royal College of Anaesthetists sets a ninety question negatively-marked multiple choice examination (MCQ) as the first hurdle in its final fellowship examination. This mode of examination is selected because it is believed to be a cost-effective means of comparing the performance of a large number of candidates against the performance of cohorts from previous years. It is regarded as an objective measure of breadth of knowledge with questions representative of the entire syllabus.

The minimum requirement to move on to the *viva* phase of the examination is a '1+' but only 14% of those holding a '1+' from the MCQ will pass overall. You should be aiming for a '2' in the MCQ. 70% of these candidates will go on to pass the FRCA at that sitting. The pass mark required to achieve a '2' probably lies between 46–53% but will vary slightly from year to year based on the performance of the year's cohort on a number of previously used discriminator or moderator questions.

Strategies for success

Two factors will determine whether you pass this negatively-marked multiple-choice examination:

1. How much do you know?
2. How many questions will you answer?

Experience, training and the effectiveness of your revision strategies will determine how much you know on the day. This is the 'objective' bit. Your personality and confidence will subjectively influence your decision about how many questions you then label 'true' or 'false' during the test, based on your fear of losing marks for incorrect responses.

The **QBase** system will help you to identify your strengths and weaknesses.

Use it as a tool to target your revision. There is no substitute for hitting the books before sitting the FRCA, but it is important that your revision schedule covers all of the syllabus in enough depth to answer questions on it. We suggest that you use the 'review questions' option after setting yourself a test. Pick out those questions where you scored less than '3' and have a second look at them. The notes section in this book has been significantly expanded so that you can identify where and why you went wrong. Follow up on the questions where you performed badly and specifically target your revision to these areas of weakness so that you use your time effectively to increase your breadth of knowledge.

Although nobody can tell you with accuracy how many questions you should answer in the real FRCA examination, our studies have shown conclusively that candidates cannot accurately identify correct responses with 100% success. Out of every ten answers that most candidates feel absolutely certain about, only nine will actually be correct. This means that with negative marking you will at best be getting 80% overall, even if you felt you were certain about the answers to all of the questions! To pass the FRCA examination you need to answer enough questions to get more than about 50% overall. Candidates who answer less than 80% of the paper (72 questions, or 360 of the 450 leaves) will find it difficult to achieve this pass mark. Try it yourself!

The problem is that you just don't know how well or badly you are really doing until the paper is marked, so a 'calculated' approach to the number of questions answered is very dangerous. We have both met candidates who have failed the exam in the past with spectacularly good 'hit' rates in terms of accuracy of their answers, but they simply answered too few questions overall to reach the pass mark.

Of even more interest is the finding that most candidates improve their score by guessing. This seems counter-intuitive in the context of a negatively-marked MCQ but is almost invariably true. Statistically, a negatively-marked examination is designed to NULLIFY, not penalise, the effects of guessing. Answer all of the questions in an MCQ exam set in Ancient Greek for instance, and your score will probably be zero. Any knowledge you bring to bear on the test will start to skew your score in a positive direction, and this is indeed what happens in practice. As a trainee approaching the Final FRCA, you will be assimilating information from an enormous range of sources. Some of this information will be categorised so that you can recall it at will. Other facts will seem right to you, but you will have no idea where the information came from. These hunches or 'guesses' are probably based on sound revision and are often worth following. Again, try it yourself. The **QBase** system allows you to include or exclude these labelled 'guesses' so that you may examine their effects on your overall score.

Finally, we wish you success in the examination. Work hard but make sure that you pass or fail on your own merits... not because you failed to tell the examiners what you knew!

Andrew McIndoe
Edward Hammond
September 2005

List of Abbreviations

AAGBI	Association of Anaesthetists of Great Britain and Ireland
ACE	angiotensin converting enzyme
ACEI	angiotensin converting enzyme inhibitor
ACT	activated clotting time
ACTH	adrenocorticotropic hormone
ADH	anti-diuretic hormone
AFP	alpha-fetoprotein
AG	anion gap
ALS algorithm	advanced life support algorithm
AMPA	aminohydroxy-methylisoxazole-propionic acid
APL valve	adjustable pressure-limiting valve
APTT	activated partial thromboplastin time
ARDS	adult respiratory distress syndrome
ARF	acute renal failure
ASA	American Society of Anesthesiologists
ASD	atrial septal defect
AST	aspartate aminotransferase
ATP	adenosine triphosphate
BiPAP	bilevel positive airway pressure
BMI	body mass index
'BURP' manoeuvre	backward, upward, rightward pressure on the thyroid cartilage
CABG	coronary artery bypass grafting
CBF	cerebral blood flow
CCK	cholecystokinin
CF	cystic fibrosis
CFTR	cystic fibrosis transmembrane conductance regulator
CGRP	calcitonin gene-related peptide
CI	cardiac index
$CMRO_2$	cerebral metabolic rate
CMV	controlled mechanical ventilation
CoHb	carboxyhaemoglobin
COPD	chronic obstructive pulmonary disease
CPAP	continuous positive airway pressure
CPD	citrate-phosphate-dextrose
CRF	chronic renal failure
CSF	cerebrospinal fluid
CT	computed tomography
CVA	cerebrovascular accident
CVP	central venous pressure

DDAVP	1-deamino-8-D-arginine vasopressin, desmopressin
DIC	disseminated intravascular coagulation
DLT	double-lumen tube
ECG	electrocardiogram
ECMO	extracorporeal membrane oxygenation
ECT	electroconvulsive therapy
EEG	electroencephalogram
EMD	electromechanical dissociation
ERCP	endoscopic retrograde cholangio-pancreaticography
ERP	endoscopic retrograde pancreaticography
ERV	expiratory reserve volume
$EtCO_2$	end expired carbon dioxide concentration
ETT	endotracheal tube
FDP	fibrinogen degradation products
FES	Fat embolism syndrome
FEV_1	forced expiratory volume in one second
FFP	fresh frozen plasma
FGF	fresh gas flow
FiO_2	inspired oxygen concentration
FRC	functional residual capacity
FSH	follicle-stimulating hormone
FVC	forced vital capacity
GA	general anaesthesia
GABA	gamma-aminobutyric acid
GBS	Guillain Barre syndrome
GCS	Glasgow Coma Score
GFR	glomerular filtration rate
GH	growth hormone
HFJV	high-frequency jet ventilation
HIAA	5-hydroxyindole acetic acid
HIV	human immunodeficiency virus
HOT	hypertension optimal treatment
HPA	hypothalmic-pituitary-adrenal
ICP	intracranial pressure
IL-1	interleukin-1
INR	International Normalised Ratio
ISAP	International Association for the Study of Pain
IVC	inferior vena cava
IVRA	intravenous regional anaesthesia
JW	Jehovah's witnesses
kPa	partial pressure

LA	local anaesthetic
LBBB	left bundle branch block
LDH	lactate dehydrogenase
LH	luteinizing hormone
LMA	laryngeal mask airway
LPS	lipopolysaccharide
LSCS	lower segment caesarean section
LSD	lysergic acid diethylamide
LVEDP	left ventricular end-diastolic pressure
LVF	left ventricular failure
MAC	minimum alveolar concentration
MAPP	minimum alveolar partial pressure
MBC	maximum breathing capacity
MDMA (Ecstasy)	"3,4-methylenedioxymethamphetamine"
MG	myasthenia gravis
MH	malignant hyperthermia
MI	myocardial infarction
MND	motor neurone disease
MODS	multiple organ dysfunction syndrome
MONA therapy	Morphine/diamorphine, Oxygen, Nitroglycerine, Aspirin
MRI	magnetic resonance imaging
N&V	nausea and vomiting
NADH	nicotinamide adenine dinucleotide
NADPH	nicotinamide adenine dinucleotide phosphate
Nd-YAG laser	neodymium-doped yttrium-aluminium-garnet laser
NEC	necrotising enterocolitis
NMDA	N-methyl-D-aspartate
NMJ	neuromuscular junction
NNT	number needed to treat
NSAID	non-steroidal anti-inflammatory drugs
OAA	Obstetric Anaesthetists' Association
$PaCO_2$	arterial carbon dioxide tension
PAF	platelet-activating factor
PaO_2	arterial oxygen tension
PAP	positive airway pressure
PCP	pneumocystis carinii pneumonia
PCWP	pulmonary capillary wedge pressure
PDA	patent ductus arteriosus
PEA	pulseless electrical activity
PEEP	positive end expiratory pressure
PRB	plasma-reduced blood
PT	prothrombin time

PVR	peripheral vascular resistance
RV	residual volume
RWMA	regional wall motion abnormalities
SA node	sinoatrial node
SAG-M	saline, adenine, glucose and mannitol
SI	Systeme Internationale
SIMV	synchronised intermittent mandatory ventilation
SIRS	systemic inflammatory response syndrome
SLE	systemic lupus erythematosus
SvO_2	mixed venous oxygen saturation
SVR	systemic vascular resistance
TEG	thromboelastograph
TIA	transient ischaemic attack
TIMI	thrombolysis in myocardial infarction
TNF	tumour necrosis factor
TOE	trans-oesophageal echocardiography
TSH	thyroid-stimulating hormone
TURP	transurethral resection of the prostate
U-D interval	uterine incision-to-delivery interval
V/Q	ventilation/perfusion
vCJD	variant Creutzfeldt-Jakob disease
Vdss	steady state volume of distribution
VSD	ventricular septal defect
WBC	white blood cell

Section 1 – Questions

Q 1. Concerning anaesthetic management of the obese patient

A. Patients are regarded as obese with a body mass index >30
B. Metabolism of halothane is greater compared to non-obese patients
C. For operations of normal time duration, recovery from volatile agents is increased
D. The laryngeal aperture is more likely to be high and anterior
E. Peripheral nerve stimulation to test neuromuscular blockade is identical to non-obese individuals

Q 2. Tourniquets

A. Lower limb tourniquets should be inflated to 200 mmHg
B. Tourniquet pain can be prevented by sympathetic blockade
C. The cuff width should exceed half the diameter of the limb
D. Soft padding should always be used beneath a tourniquet
E. Tourniquet pain is mediated by C fibres

Q 3. Concerning the Goldman cardiac risk index

A. It scores patients undergoing cardiac surgery
B. Severe aortic stenosis is the highest individual scorer
C. Not all high-risk patients are identified
D. It has a low sensitivity
E. Age >70 years is a risk factor

Q 4. Headache following spinal anaesthesia

A. Is classically frontal or occipital
B. Is more common in women
C. Is more likely with paramedian than midline approach
D. Is more common in pregnant than non-pregnant patients
E. Nearly always resolves without therapy in time

Q 5. **Cricoid pressure**

A. Is also known as Sellick's manoeuvre
B. Is digital pressure on the cricothyroid membrane
C. Involves the use of 20 N of force
D. Is performed using thumb and middle fingers only
E. Should be maintained until the endotracheal tube cuff is inflated if the patient vomits during induction

Q 6. **During intravenous regional anaesthesia (IVRA) or Bier's block for surgery on the upper limb**

A. A large bore IV cannula should be sited
B. Inflation of a distal tourniquet prior to the proximal one reduces tourniquet pain during the procedure
C. Prilocaine 2% is the preferred local anaesthetic agent with the safest therapeutic index
D. The principal contraindication is systolic hypertension
E. Tourniquet deflation should occur immediately the procedure is finished to reduce ischaemic side effects

Q 7. **The following are signs of adequate preoperative preparation of a patient who is to undergo excision of a phaeochromocytoma**

A. Nasal congestion
B. Decreased frequency of bowel motions
C. Orthostatic hypotension
D. Decreased body weight
E. Increased haematocrit

Q 8. **Concerning diabetes mellitus in pregnancy**

A. Oral hypoglycaemic agents should be replaced by subcutaneous insulin in the second trimester
B. Tight glycaemic control is mandatory
C. An intravenous insulin infusion should be commenced to cover labour
D. Urine glucose should be tested regularly to guide insulin requirements
E. The risk of foetal acidosis during labour is a contraindication to the use of epidural analgesia

Concerning blood products for transfusion

A. Plasma-reduced blood (PRB) consists of red cells suspended in an artificial nutrient solution
B. CPD blood (citrate, dextrose, phosphate) cooled to 4°C can be stored for an almost indefinite period
C. Cryoprecipitate is rich in fibrinogen
D. The half-life of transfused platelets is about 4 days
E. Fresh frozen plasma (FFP) must be ABO blood group compatible with the recipient

Q 10. **Concerning the anaesthetic management of a child requiring the removal of an inhaled foreign body**

A. Hyperinflation of the lung distal to a 'ball-valve' obstruction is best seen with a chest radiograph taken on inspiration
B. The maximum dose of lignocaine spray for anaesthetising the larynx and trachea is 4–5 mg/kg
C. The Stortz bronchoscope has an attachment for the anaesthetic breathing system
D. The Negus bronchoscope is a flexible bronchoscope
E. Suxamethonium is relatively contraindicated

Q 11. **The following can occur**

A. Supraventricular tachycardia during extracorporeal shock wave lithotripsy
B. Seizures with cerebral angiography
C. Indirect observation of a patient during radiation therapy
D. Burns with MRI
E. Hypothermia during computed tomography

Q 12. **Patients with sickle cell trait**

A. Have protection against Plasmodium Falciparum
B. Have approximately 40% HbSS
C. May have a sickle crisis if exposed to hypoxia
D. Have a positive sickle test
E. Often get aseptic necrosis of the femoral head

Q 13. When preparing for awake intubation

A. A maximum of 6 mg/kg cocaine may be used topically

B. The epiglottis may be anaesthetised using a superior laryngeal nerve block

C. During trans-tracheal injection it is best to ask the patient to breathe in before injection

D. Nebulised lignocaine can be used as the only local anaesthetic

E. After using a fibreoptic instrument, disinfectant should be passed through it to clean it

Q 14. Anaphylactic reactions

A. Are type A adverse reactions

B. Are most frequently characterised by a decrease in blood pressure

C. Blood for serum tryptase levels should be taken immediately after treatment with adrenaline

D. Future investigation of the patient should involve skin testing with all anaesthetic drugs used including volatiles

E. Immediate treatment includes 100 μg of adrenaline (epinephrine) given intramuscularly

Q 15. The following are true

A. The fresh gas flow runs through the outer tube of a coaxial Mapleson D breathing system

B. A leak in the inner tube of a Bain will cause the bag to deflate

C. A fresh gas flow of 4.2 L/min will produce normocapnia in a 60-kg ventilated patient using a Mapleson D circuit

D. A Mapleson A requires a fresh gas flow of at least 70 ml/kg/min for controlled ventilation

E. There is no way to humidify the fresh gas flow with the Mapleson F circuit

Q 16. Concerning the cranial nerves

A. The third nerve supplies levator palpebrae superioris

B. The dilated pupil seen with raised intracranial pressure is due to compression of the sixth cranial nerve

C. Taste from the anterior two thirds of the tongue is transmitted (via the chorda tympani) in the seventh cranial nerve
D. Sensation from the tip of the nose is carried in nerve fibres that pass through the foramen rotundum
E. Ramsay Hunt syndrome results in a small irregular pupil that accommodates but does not react to light

Q 17. Anticholinesterases

A. Containing a quaternary ammonium group are more likely to cause CNS effects
B. Prolong SA and AV node conduction time
C. Cause pupillary constriction
D. Relieve bronchospasm
E. Increase intraocular pressure

Q 18. Considering the renin-angiotensin system

A. Spironolactone is an antagonist at aldosterone receptors
B. Angiotensin stimulates the release of aldosterone
C. Angiotensin converting enzyme (ACE) inhibitors suppress the release of aldosterone
D. Spironolactone is a potassium-sparing diuretic
E. Mortality in severe heart failure treated by ACE inhibitors is improved by adding spironolactone

Q 19. Halothane

A. Has a blood gas solubility of 1.9
B. Is metabolised to a greater extent than enflurane or isoflurane
C. Causes bronchoconstriction
D. Is more negatively inotropic than enflurane
E. Causes a reflex tachycardia

Q 20. Desflurane

A. Has a blood gas solubility of 0.6
B. Has a MAC value that is less than that of cyclopropane
C. Is approximately 2% metabolised
D. Has a boiling point of 39°C
E. Has a lower molecular weight than sevoflurane

Q 21. Concerning intracranial pressure (ICP)

A. Lumbar puncture raising the height of a CSF manometer to 15 cm is abnormal

B. Tonsillar (cerebellar) herniation causes ipsilateral pupillary dilatation

C. Lundberg B pressure waves may be a normal finding

D. The effect of hypocapnia-induced cerebral vasoconstriction is maintained after 12 h

E. Intracranial pressure monitoring is of use in fulminant hepatic failure

Q 22. Concerning the blood supply of the kidney

A. The renal arteries divide into arterioles then capillaries then arterioles then vasa recta

B. The afferent arterioles are more sensitive than the efferent to angiotensin II

C. Administration of non-steroidal anti-inflammatory drugs (NSAIDs) to normal kidneys reduces glomerular filtration rate (GFR) by 20%

D. Symptomatic uraemia usually develops when the GFR is about 15 ml/min

E. In the normal young adult renal blood flow is about 1,200 ml per min

Q 23. Concerning pulmonary function tests

A. FEV_1/FVC of 50% suggests a restrictive defect

B. In obstructive disease, the total lung capacity is typically abnormally large

C. FEV_1 is reduced by reducing airway resistance

D. FRC can be measured using helium dilution

E. Pendelluft may result in lung areas with long time constants filling during expiration

Q 24. Carbon Dioxide

A. Diffuses rapidly across cell membranes

B. Forms carbonic acid in erythrocytes

C. Is displaced from haemoglobin by oxygen

D. The value of oxygen uptake/carbon dioxide output is the respiratory quotient

E. The total amount dissolved in body tissues is approximately 12 l

Q 25. The following mechanisms are involved in peripheral neuropathic pain

A. Spontaneous activity in large myelinated A fibres

B. Schwann cell de-differentiation

C. Phosphorylation of the AMPA receptor

D. Increased production of cholecystokinin

E. Sprouting of sympathetic nerve terminals in the dorsal horn

Q 26. Concerning pain pathways

A. C fibres are myelinated

B. C fibres are involved in slow pain transmission

C. Both A delta and C fibres synapse in the substantia gelatinosa

D. The principal ascending paths are the spinothalamic tracts

E. Nerve fibres for temperature follow the same pathways as fibres for pain

Q 27. In aortic stenosis

A. The murmur is classically mid-systolic

B. If symptomatic, is associated with an average survival of <2–3 years

C. A transvalvular pressure gradient <50 mmHg or a valve area >1.0 cm^2 excludes severe stenosis

D. Atrial contraction can contribute 40% of left ventricular end diastolic volume

E. Nitrate therapy is contraindicated

Q 28. Concerning respiratory tract tumours

A. Small cell carcinoma is the commonest type

B. Alveolar cell carcinoma is not related to smoking

C. Squamous cell carcinomas may cavitate

D. Unilateral ptosis, miosis and enophthalmos are present in Horner's syndrome

E. Adenocarcinomas usually present with obstruction of a main bronchus

Q 29. Concerning patients with portal hypertension

A. The portal venous pressure in normal humans is about 17 mmHg

B. β-adrenergic antagonists reduce portal venous pressure

C. Terlipressin, a synthetic analogue of vasopressin, is devoid of coronary side effects

D. Pharmacological therapy with octreotide is superior to emergency endoscopic management of acutely bleeding oesophageal varices

E. Portal hypertension may be a consequence of constrictive pericarditis

Q 30. Serum cardiac troponin I and troponin T

A. Are undetectable in healthy individuals

B. Are exclusively derived from the myocardial contractile apparatus

C. Can be used to screen for re-infarction

D. Are elevated in renal failure

E. Are elevated following pulmonary embolus

Q 31. Congenital heart disease

A. Coarctation of the aorta is the commonest congenital heart lesion in Down's syndrome

B. Eisenmenger's syndrome may occur in patients with a VSD

C. Atrial septal defects are usually associated with right bundle branch block and right axis deviation

D. Coarctation of the aorta is usually proximal to the insertion of the ductus arteriosus

E. Cyanotic 'spells' in children with Fallot's tetralogy should be treated with 21% oxygen

Q 32. In paediatric practice

A. The most frequent site of metastases of a Wilm's tumour (nephroblastoma) is the lung

B. Marfan's syndrome is inherited in an autosomal dominant pattern

C. Children with Prader-Willi syndrome are likely to be hypotonic and cachectic

D. Patients with central core disease frequently present with congenital dislocation of the hip

E. Maternal treatment with carbimazole may cause goitre in newborn infants

Q 33. Hereditary angioneurotic oedema (C1-esterase deficiency)

A. Classically affects the lungs

B. Causes life-threatening upper airway obstruction during dental extractions

C. Responds well to steroids

D. Responds well to adrenaline

E. Is a contraindication to regional anaesthesia

Q 34. Accepted techniques of anaesthesia for carotid artery surgery

A. Include the use of just a cervical plexus block

B. Include controlled hypotension to reduce blood loss

C. Utilise intravenous glucose infusion to provide cerebroprotection

D. Utilise hyperventilation to increase cerebral blood flow

E. Include carotid sinus infiltration with local anaesthetic solution to prevent hypotension

Q 35. Patients with Marfan's syndrome

A. Are more likely to need ophthalmic surgery than the normal population

B. Are prone to pneumothoraces

C. Are susceptible to bacterial endocarditis

D. Are at higher risk of difficult intubation than the normal population

E. Are at higher risk of death in pregnancy than the normal population

Q 36. The following statements are correct with relation to surgical metabolic derangements

A. Pyloric stenosis is associated with a hypochloraemic metabolic alkalosis

B. A chronic plasma potassium of <3.0 mmol/L is associated with a total body deficit of 200–300 mmol

Exam 1

Questions

C. Pancreatic fistulae are associated with metabolic acidosis
D. Fat malabsorption is associated with hyperoxaluria
E. Secondary hyperparathyroidism is associated with hypercalcaemia

Q 37. In gastrointestinal surgery

A. The trans-hiatal approach to oesophagectomy is often associated with atrial compression
B. The Ivor Lewis oesophagectomy involves a left thoracotomy
C. The Nissen fundoplication procedure can be performed laparoscopically
D. A Whipple's procedure involves partial gastrectomy, duodenectomy, partial pancreatectomy and distal choledochectomy
E. Only 10% of colorectal cancers are found in the sigmoid and rectum

Q 38. In patients for hepatic surgery

A. The Childs' classification is a measure of hepatic encephalopathy
B. The renin-angiotensin system is activated in patients with advanced liver disease
C. Patients with advanced liver disease typically have a low cardiac output and high systemic vascular resistance
D. Urine sodium concentration is >100 mmol/L in those patients with hepatorenal syndrome
E. Factor 7 is usually reduced in liver disease

Q 39. Concerning acute spinal cord injury

A. There are usually 2 anterior spinal arteries and 1 posterior spinal artery supplying the spinal cord with blood
B. Hyperglycaemia is associated with a worse neurological outcome
C. Patients receiving methylprednisolone within 8 h of injury have better motor and sensory function in the long term
D. The areflexic phase of injury usually ends between 4 weeks and 3 months afterwards
E. Suxamethonium becomes safe to use again after the areflexic phase

Q 40. Cement use during orthopaedic surgery

    A. Acts as a glue
    B. The odour of the volatile monomer is a biohazard
    C. Is more effective if a hypotensive anaesthetic technique is used
    D. The rate of hypotension caused can be reduced by washing out the bone cavity with normal saline
    E. May be directly cardiotoxic

Q 41. Concerning direct measurement of arterial blood pressure

    A. Optimal damping offers the most rapid response of the output waveform to change without amplitude overshoot
    B. When the damping coefficient equals 1.0, the damping is said to be optimal
    C. For faithful reproduction of the shape of the arterial waveform the first 10 harmonics of the heart rate are required
    D. An overdamped system may lead to the recording of an artefactually high pulse pressure
    E. Critical damping is said to occur when the system just fails to oscillate in response to change

Q 42. Concerning trans-oesophageal echocardiography (TOE)

    A. TOE is an insensitive monitor of air embolism
    B. Regional wall motion abnormalities indicate myocardial ischaemia
    C. Regional wall motion abnormalities indicate tethered myocardium
    D. Ejection fraction can be monitored continuously
    E. The appearance of regional wall motion abnormalities may represent normal variability

Q 43. Concerning coagulation studies

    A. The prothrombin time (PT) tests the extrinsic and common coagulation pathways
    B. The activated clotting time (ACT) normal value is 30–40 s
    C. The bleeding time is normally 2–9 min

Exam 1

Questions

D. The thromboelastogram gives little information about the speed of formation and the quality of clot
E. The activated partial thromboplastin time (APTT) is performed using plasma, calcium, brain extract and phospholipid

Q 44. When assessing degree of residual neuromuscular blockade

A. Normal tidal volume may be achieved with 80% receptor occupancy
B. A head lift can be sustained with 75% receptor occupancy
C. Train of four count will detect 50% receptor occupancy
D. A normal handgrip is possible with 50% receptor occupancy
E. Sustained tetanus at 100-Hz stimulation indicates complete reversal

Q 45. In the ECG

A. A Q wave in V6 is normal
B. A Q wave in III is a normal variant
C. Left atrial hypertrophy causes peaked P waves
D. Digoxin causes downsloping ST depression and T wave inversion
E. Wolff-Parkinson-White syndrome is caused by an abnormal myocardial connection between atrium and ventricle

Q 46. Regarding temperature measurement

A. The Bourdon gauge is really a device for measuring pressure
B. Infrared tympanic membrane thermometers are in common clinical use
C. The thermocouple is an electrical technique for measuring temperature
D. The Seebeck effect may be utilised
E. Electrical temperature-measuring probes have a heat capacity proportional to their size

Q 47. In Fat Embolism syndrome

A. Isolated respiratory insufficiency is common
B. A characteristic petechial rash affects the upper extremities
C. A left ventricular strain pattern is frequently observed on a 12-lead ECG

D. Deterioration in arterial oxygen tension precedes chest radiographic changes

E. Thrombocytopaenia and hypocalcaemia are pathognomonic of the condition

Q 48. The following treatment strategies are appropriate in cardiogenic shock

A. Intra-aortic balloon counterpulsation pump

B. Surgery

C. α-adrenergic receptor agonists

D. Sodium nitroprusside

E. Amiodarone

Q 49. Appropriate management of an acute myocardial infarction should include

A. Thrombolytic therapy if ST elevation of 0.1 mV is present in 2 adjacent chest leads

B. Aspirin 300 mg orally

C. Opioid analgesia if the patient has chest pain

D. Sublingual nifedipine if the patient is hypertensive

E. Thrombolytic therapy if aortic dissection is suspected

Q 50. The following facts about tetanus are true

A. *Clostridium tetani* is an obligate anaerobic, spore-bearing gram-negative bacillus

B. Natural immunity to tetanus follows infection

C. The clinical effects of tetanus are caused by the toxin tetanolysin

D. C. tetani is an invasive organism that is non-communicable from person to person

E. Toxin binds to γ-aminobutyric acid (GABA) terminals in the brain

Q 51. The following complications are known to occur in severe sepsis

A. Perivascular thromboembolism

B. Hypoglycaemia

C. Hyperglycaemia

D. Negative nitrogen balance

E. Gastrointestinal haemorrhage

Q 52. In hypothermia

 A. Core temperature will be <35°C
 B. A 'J' wave may be seen at the junction of the P wave and the QRS complex
 C. Renal blood flow initially increases
 D. Respiratory drive ceases at a core temperature of around 30°C
 E. Asystole usually occurs below 20°C

Q 53. Botulism

 A. Is caused by a spore-forming gram-negative bacillus
 B. Is mostly caused by the contamination of wounds with soil-borne organisms
 C. Is caused by the effects of an exotoxin
 D. Prevents acetylcholine release from nerve endings
 E. Increases lower limb deep tendon reflexes

Q 54. In acute severe asthma which requires mechanical ventilation

 A. Intrinsic PEEP is measured at the end of inspiration
 B. Increasing ventilatory rate can cause an increase in pulmonary hyperinflation
 C. Hypotension on initiating ventilation should be treated with fluid loading
 D. Lactic acidosis is a recognised complication of parenteral β-agonist administration
 E. Neuromuscular-blocking drugs cause myopathy in ventilated asthmatics

Q 55. The following modes of ventilation may be applied to non-intubated patients

 A. CMV
 B. BiPAP
 C. CPAP
 D. SIMV
 E. Pressure support ventilation

Q 56. In carbon monoxide poisoning

 A. CO has 250 times the affinity for haemoglobin than O_2
 B. Pulse oximetry and PaO_2 become inaccurate

C. CO levels of 6% are compatible with a smoker

D. Dissociation of carboxyhaemoglobin is increased by administration of 100% O_2 by simple facemask

E. CO tends to displace CO_2 molecules to form carboxyhaemoglobin

Q 57. Concerning pneumonia

A. *H. influenzae* is the commonest cause of community-acquired pneumonia in previously well patients

B. Streptococcal pneumonia often follows a viral infection

C. Mycoplasma pneumonia often occurs in epidemics

D. Cold agglutinins occur in approximately 5% of patients with mycoplasma pneumonia

E. Rose spots may occur in patients with *Chlamydia Psittaci* pneumonia

Q 58. The following cause a metabolic acidosis

A. Salicylate poisoning

B. Guillain-Barre syndrome

C. Acetazolamide administration

D. Diarrhoea

E. Cyanide poisoning

Q 59. A low plasma urea : creatinine ratio occurs in

A. Liver failure

B. Patients on diuretic therapy

C. Patients on corticosteroid therapy

D. Cardiac failure

E. Pregnancy

Q 60. The following statements relating to perioperative nutritional support are correct

A. Fat solutions are non-irritants and may be administered by a peripheral intravenous infusion

B. Carbohydrate calories are more efficient than lipid calories

C. 20% of the total energy can be given as protein sources

D. Essential amino acids should constitute at least 50% of the total nitrogen content of any given feed

E. Arginine is an amino acid that facilitates nitrogen transport and is the major fuel for enterocytes

Q 1.   Concerning anaesthesia for neurosurgery

- **A.** Nitrous oxide increases cerebral blood flow
- **B.** Mannitol may increase bleeding
- **C.** Steroids given to head-injured patients are able to control intracranial pressure
- **D.** Phenytoin should be given to a patient with an acute subdural haematoma
- **E.** Dehydration assists in the control of intracranial pressure

Q 2.   During magnetic resonance imaging

- **A.** It is noisy
- **B.** There is a risk of microshock through pulmonary artery catheters
- **C.** Looped fibreoptic cables lead to problems with induced currents
- **D.** Non-invasive blood pressure measurement is impossible
- **E.** The magnetic field interferes with capnometry

Q 3.   Hartmann's solution 500 ml contains

- **A.** 5 mmol of potassium
- **B.** 131 mmol of chloride
- **C.** 1 mmol calcium
- **D.** 131 mmol of sodium
- **E.** 29 mmol of lactate

Q 4.   Concerning an inhaled foreign body

- **A.** Most objects lodge in the left main bronchus
- **B.** CXR may reveal unilateral overinflation
- **C.** Positive pressure ventilation should be avoided
- **D.** Nitrous oxide should not be used
- **E.** Removal is usually achieved by flexible bronchoscopy

Q 5. **Concerning anaesthesia for laparoscopic cholecystectomy**

A. The stomach should be aspirated of contents prior to the commencement of surgery
B. Venous return may be reduced
C. Aortic compression can lead to hypotension
D. There is a risk of explosion if laparoscopic diathermy is used with CO_2 as the insufflating gas
E. Gas flow rates should not exceed 1L/min

Q 6. **Concerning anaesthesia for patients with Down's syndrome**

A. Congenital heart disease is common
B. Atlantoaxial instability occurs
C. Hypertonia is common
D. The incidence of difficult intubation is increased
E. The syndrome results from trisomy 23

Q 7. **Regarding the anaesthetic management of a patient with essential hypertension**

A. Elective surgery should be postponed in the presence of a repeated blood pressure reading of 180/110 mmHg
B. The cardiac output is considerably greater than in an age-matched normotensive patient
C. Preoperative optimisation of blood pressure greatly reduces the subsequent risk of stroke occurring in the perioperative period
D. Global myocardial ischaemia is common
E. The slope of the downstroke of the arterial waveform reflects the compliance of the systemic vascular bed

Q 8. **The following are recognised complications of lower segment caesarean section (LSCS) performed under regional anaesthesia**

A. Amniotic fluid embolism
B. Air embolism
C. Delayed respiratory depression
D. Mendelson's syndrome
E. Poor condition of the neonate at birth when the induction of anaesthesia to delivery interval exceeds 15 min

Q 9. In haemophilia 'A'

A. At least 30% factor VIII activity is required for surgery
B. There is no platelet defect
C. The prothrombin time is abnormal but the partial thromboplastin time is normal
D. Males and females are affected equally
E. Postoperative bleeding is decreased by tranexamic acid due to its inhibitory action on fibrinolysis

Q 10. Regarding perioperative fluid balance in paediatric practice

A. Maintenance fluid should include glucose in an otherwise fit neonate
B. Intravenous infusions administered to children under 5 years of age should routinely be supplemented with potassium
C. 10 ml/kg/h is the intraoperative fluid volume requirement of a healthy child weighing up to 10 kg
D. 0.3–0.5 ml/kg/h of urine production is consistent with adequate hydration
E. Transfusion with blood can be safely deferred until over 10% of the circulating blood volume has been lost

Q 11. Effects of electroconvulsive therapy (ECT) include

A. Elevated intraocular pressure
B. Decreased cerebral blood flow
C. Hypertension initially followed later by hypotension
D. Increased intragastric pressure
E. Arrhythmias

Q 12. At high altitudes as compared to sea level

A. A higher partial pressure of anaesthetic agent is required to produce anaesthesia
B. A higher set concentration of desflurane is required to produce anaesthesia
C. Alveolar concentration of anaesthetic agent will need to be higher to achieve the same degree of anaesthesia
D. The Fluotec Mark 2 vaporiser is unsuitable for clinical use
E. A higher set concentration of halothane is required to produce anaesthesia

Q 13. Anaesthetic considerations for phaeochromocytoma

A. Blood pressure stabilises after tumour removal
B. Preoperative preparation should commence with an oral β-antagonist
C. Cardiomyopathy can occur
D. Magnesium sulphate should not be used to control hypertension per-operatively
E. Only adrenaline (epinephrine) and noradrenaline (norepinephrine) are secreted

Q 14. Concerning the anaesthetic management of a pre-eclamptic patient

A. Total body clearance of amide local anaesthetics is prolonged
B. Intubation can be more difficult due to a swollen tongue
C. Higher doses of vasopressor are required in hypotension associated with regional blockade
D. The action of non-depolarising neuromuscular blockers is prolonged with the concurrent use of magnesium sulphate
E. Epidural anaesthesia does not alter placental perfusion

Q 15. The following associations are correct concerning endobronchial tubes

A. Carlens tube has no carinal hook
B. Robertshaw tube is only available in a left-sided version
C. Bryce-Smith tube has a carinal hook
D. Left-sided tubes are usually preferred even for most right-sided surgery
E. Brompton Pallister tube is passed into the right main bronchus

Q 16. The aortic and pulmonary valves

A. Have three cusps
B. Give rise to the second and third heart sounds
C. Are thinner than the atrioventricular valves
D. Are semilunar valves
E. Are supported by chordae tendineae

Q 17. The following antihypertensives are correctly paired with their primary site of action

A. Thiazide diuretics : distal convoluted tubule
B. β-blockers : renin release
C. Prazosin : α_2-adrenoreceptor
D. ACE inhibitors : conversion of angiotensinogen
E. Calcium channel blockers : L-type calcium channels in the vascular smooth muscle

Q 18. 5-HT$_3$ antagonists

A. Cause dose-related extrapyramidal effects
B. Improve age-related memory impairment
C. Are all prokinetic
D. Diminish the 'high' associated with heroin abuse
E. Are anxiolytic

Q 19. Enflurane

A. Typically depresses the respiratory rate
B. Causes a reflex tachycardia
C. Commonly causes an increase in bronchial secretions
D. Causes hypotension mainly by its negative inotropic effects
E. Has a blood gas solubility of 2.5

Q 20. Comparing desflurane and isoflurane

A. Desflurane is more stable than isoflurane
B. Desflurane is less soluble in blood than isoflurane
C. Desflurane exerts a greater degree of circulatory depression than isoflurane
D. Desflurane is metabolised to a greater extent than isoflurane
E. Desflurane is more pungent than isoflurane

Q 21. Concerning neuromuscular transmission

A. Adenosine and calcitonin gene-related peptide (CGRP) are transmitters at the neuromuscular junction
B. During fasciculation muscle fibres contract synchronously
C. The presence of the nerve fibre determines the type of acetylcholine receptor expressed by the muscle

D. Pancuronium increases release of noradrenaline from sympathetic nerve terminals

E. Tetanic fade and 'train-of-four' phenomena result from presynaptic acetylcholine receptor antagonism

Q 22. Concerning the foetal circulation

A. The saturation of foetal arterial blood is approximately 65%

B. The saturation of the blood in the umbilical vein is 80%

C. Prostaglandin E1 is used to aid closure of a patent ductus arteriosus (PDA)

D. The resuscitation of an initially apnoeic neonate should begin with assisted breaths at 40–50/min

E. The placenta protects the foetus from the transfer of local anaesthetic drugs

Q 23. Stimulation of the parasympathetic nervous system causes

A. Mydriasis

B. Urinary sphincter relaxation

C. Bronchial smooth muscle relaxation

D. Gall bladder contraction

E. GI tract sphincter relaxation

Q 24. Blood pressure

A. In the dorsalis pedis artery is often higher than in the aorta

B. Most of the decrease in blood pressure between the arterial and venous system occurs in the capillaries

C. Pulsus paradoxus is an exaggerated decrease in systolic blood pressure during expiration

D. Is altered by atrial distension

E. Is controlled by the Traube–Hering reflex

Q 25. The following transmitters are present in the dorsal horn as part of the descending (inhibitory) pain control system

A. Bradykinin

B. Noradrenaline

C. Serotonin
D. Substance P
E. GABA

Q 26. Concerning back pain

A. 95% of lumbar vertebral disc herniation occurs at the L4/L5 and L5/S1 levels
B. Pain is produced by contact of the prolapsed disc with the nerve root
C. L5/S1 disc herniation produces pain in the buttocks, posterior thigh, anterolateral lower limb, medial foot and great toe
D. Up to 20% of the asymptomatic population demonstrate disc prolapse or spinal stenosis on CT or MRI scan
E. A positive straight leg raise will produce pain in the appropriate distribution at ≤60° elevation

Q 27. Patients in chronic renal failure

A. Demonstrate delayed gastric emptying
B. Commonly have a prolonged APTT
C. Commonly have a normochromic normocytic anaemia
D. Should not be given 0.9% saline
E. Are given perioperative DDAVP to improve renal function

Q 28. Concerning pulmonary hypertension

A. It is defined as a mean PAP >15 mmHg
B. A rise in $PaCO_2$ after administration of oxygen in a COPD patient is due to the decrease in hypoxic drive
C. Right ventricular hypertrophy is clinically expressed by a left parasternal heave
D. Pulmonary hypertension is a recognised consequence of congenital thoracic kyphoscoliosis
E. Type V phosphodiesterase inhibitors are useful in the management of right ventricular failure

Q 29. Chronic liver disease

A. Can be classified according to Child's criteria
B. Spontaneous bacterial peritonitis occurs in fewer than 2% of patients with ascites

C. Is associated with hypoxia

D. Is a feature of cystic fibrosis

E. Producing hepatorenal syndrome can be distinguished from hypovolaemia using urine and blood analysis

Q 30. Human Immunodeficiency Virus

A. Viral CD4 antigen is detectable in blood soon after infection

B. Contains reverse transcriptase

C. Cytomegalovirus is a common cause of eye disease

D. Seroconversion following a needlestick injury with known HIV-infected blood occurs in approximately 3% of cases

E. Kaposi's sarcoma may affect the lungs

Q 31. Concerning multiple sclerosis

A. Suxamethonium may result in hyperkalaemia

B. There is an increased incidence of epilepsy

C. There is an increased incidence of thrombocytopaenia

D. Smaller doses of non-depolarising agents may be required

E. Tremor is an early associated finding

Q 32. In motor neurone disease

A. Patients commonly present with severe muscle pain

B. Patients often have both upper and lower motor neurone signs

C. Intravenous immunoglobulin should be given as soon as possible after diagnosis

D. Cerebellar signs are common

E. Bulbar palsy may occur

Q 33. Concerning thyroid function

A. 3% of patients who have received radioactive iodine therapy for hyperthyroidism will become hypothyroid per year

B. Thyroxine and an antithyroid drug may be given for hyperthyroidism

C. Hypothyroidism is a cause of hypercholesterolaemia

D. Patients with hypothyroidism and ischaemic heart disease require urgent thyroxine therapy

E. Critical illness reduces serum tri-iodothyronine levels

Exam 2

Questions

Q 34. Concerning subarachnoid haemorrhage

- **A.** The commonest site for a berry aneurysm is the junction of the posterior communicating artery and the internal carotid
- **B.** Of patients who re-bleed, 70% will die
- **C.** The most favourable time to operate is 1 week after the first bleed
- **D.** In previously well patients, unruptured aneurysms <10 mm in diameter should be prophylactically treated
- **E.** Systolic hypertension >160 mmHg in the postoperative period should be treated

Q 35. Concerning carotid endarterectomy

- **A.** The perioperative mortality and disabling stroke rate is 7%
- **B.** A Javid shunt is equivalent to a 70% stenosis
- **C.** Regional anaesthesia has to be converted to general in approximately 2%
- **D.** Bilateral procedures result in loss of hypoxic drive
- **E.** Asymptomatic, severe (>70%) carotid stenosis should be operated on prior to coronary artery bypass grafting (CABG)

Q 36. In paediatric cardiac surgery

- **A.** Prostaglandin E1 may be used for maintaining the patency of the ductus arteriosus in patients with right to left shunts
- **B.** A Blalock-Taussig shunt is an anastamosis between pulmonary artery and subclavian vein
- **C.** The Rashkind procedure is usually performed via midline sternotomy
- **D.** Transposition of the great arteries requires a communication between the pulmonary and systemic circulation for survival
- **E.** Tetralogy of Fallot consists of ventricular septal defect, pulmonary stenosis, overriding aorta and right ventricular hypertrophy

Q 37. During TURP

- **A.** Using distilled water for irrigation leads to intravascular haemolysis
- **B.** TUR syndrome is caused by absorption of irrigating fluid through open venous sinuses

C. Severe hyponatraemia due to the TUR syndrome causes widening of the QRS complex

D. If bladder perforation occurs, it is likely to be intraperitoneal

E. Loop diuretics are a useful treatment for TUR syndrome

Q 38. Gastric cancer

A. Is associated with blood group A

B. Is the commonest site of GI cancer

C. Following resection, AFP should be monitored regularly to detect recurrence

D. Is usually an adenocarcinoma

E. Is associated with pernicious anaemia

Q 39. Concerning the formation of a tracheostomy

A. The thyroid isthmus usually covers the 2nd and 3rd tracheal rings

B. A tracheostomy should be made between the 1st and 2nd tracheal rings

C. Clinically relevant post-tracheostomy tracheal stenosis occurs in up to 8% of patients

D. A tracheostomy track has formed sufficiently to change a tube safely after 48 h

E. The incidence of complications following tracheostomy is greater after a prolonged period of endotracheal intubation

Q 40. Concerning assessment of the possibility of difficult intubation

A. The Mallampati classification is performed with the mouth at maximal opening and the tongue protruded

B. In patients with cervical disease a Mallampati class 3 view has a high positive predictive value

C. In obstetric patients a Mallampati class 3 view has a high positive predictive value

D. Applying the Mallampati test in the general surgical population allows more than half of difficult intubations to be predicted

E. In patients who cannot protrude their lower incisors to meet their upper incisors, half the direct laryngoscopies will be difficult

Q 41. The pulmonary capillary wedge pressure may not reflect left ventricular end-diastolic pressure in the following circumstances

- **A.** Right atrial myxoma
- **B.** Severe mitral stenosis
- **C.** Severe pulmonary stenosis
- **D.** High applied positive end-expiratory pressure
- **E.** If the catheter tip is in West's zone I

Q 42. When monitoring neuromuscular blockade

- **A.** Clinical monitoring of the degree of recovery is as accurate as using a nerve stimulator
- **B.** Sustained head lift (>5s) is the most reliable clinical sign of recovery of neuromuscular function
- **C.** The respiratory muscles are less sensitive to neuromuscular blockers than the small muscles of the hand
- **D.** Double burst stimulation requires two short periods of tetanic stimulation separated by 2s
- **E.** Currents of up to 6 A are required for skin electrode stimulation of peripheral nerves

Q 43. Mixed venous oxygen saturation (SvO$_2$)

- **A.** Increases in response to increased arterial saturation
- **B.** Is increased by peripheral shunting
- **C.** Rises in response to acute haemorrhage
- **D.** Rises in response to blood transfusion
- **E.** Can be measured from the inferior vena cava

Q 44. The Wright respirometer

- **A.** Is a good device for measuring tidal volumes in anaesthesia
- **B.** Is accurate for continuous flow measurement
- **C.** The electronic version is affected by moisture
- **D.** Under-reads at high volumes
- **E.** Volume measurement is achieved by monitoring the continuous rotation of a vane

Q 45. Considering inhalational anaesthetic agents

A. Critical temperature is the temperature below which a substance cannot be liquefied however much pressure is applied

B. The critical temperature of nitrous oxide is 36.5°C

C. The term 'vapour' is used to describe a substance when it exists above its critical temperature

D. The filling ratio is the mass of gas in a cylinder divided by the mass of gas it could hold if full

E. The 'pseudo-critical temperature' is that below which a gas mixture may separate into its constituents

Q 46. Regarding humidity

A. For the same mass of water vapour, relative humidity decreases with temperature

B. The hair hygrometer measures absolute humidity with a hair that reduces in length with humidity

C. The hair hygrometer is inaccurate for humidities greater than 70%

D. Regnault's hygrometer relies on the principle of the dew point

E. At normal body temperature the saturated vapour pressure of water is 6.3 kPa

Q 47. During cardiopulmonary resuscitation

A. Lignocaine (lidocaine) reduces the threshold and energy required for defibrillation

B. Bretylium is recommended in cases of refractory ventricular fibrillation

C. Sodium bicarbonate causes cerebral alkalosis

D. Potent α-adrenergic stimulants (methoxamine and phenylephrine) may be as effective as adrenaline (epinephrine)

E. Isoprenaline (isoproterenol) is an appropriate alternative to atropine for severe bradycardias

Q 48. The following statements about circulatory shock are true

A. In early shock oliguria occurs due to a reduction in glomerular filtration rate

B. A reduction in PaO_2 is an early indicator of circulatory shock

C. Neurogenic shock most commonly results from head injury
D. Hyperglycaemia is predominantly due to insulin resistance
E. Fat catabolism is inhibited

Q 49. The following statements about Acute Respiratory Distress Syndrome (ARDS) are true

A. Mortality <33%
B. Most patients die from hypoxaemia
C. Moderate to severe pulmonary dysfunction is common amongst surviving patients
D. Lung injury is homogeneous
E. Reverse ratio ventilation techniques have been shown to improve outcome

Q 50. The following therapeutic options are used during the management of tetanus

A. Clonidine
B. Magnesium
C. Metronidazole
D. Benzylpenicillin
E. Hyperbaric oxygen

Q 51. The following cytokines are thought to be involved in the aetiology of Multiple Organ Dysfunction Syndrome (MODS)

A. Tumour necrosis factor (TNF)
B. Lipopolysaccharide (LPS)
C. Platelet-activating factor (PAF)
D. Nitric oxide
E. Interleukin-1 (IL-1)

Q 52. The following statements regarding sepsis are correct

A. Diagnosis of systemic inflammatory response syndrome (SIRS) requires a white blood count of >18,000 cells/mm^3 or <400 cells/mm^3
B. Septic shock is defined as sepsis associated with organ dysfunction, hypoperfusion or hypotension
C. Interleukin-6 and interleukin-10 are anti-inflammatory

D. Interleukin-1 and interleukin-8 are proinflammatory

E. Ischaemia reperfusion injury is implicated in the inflammatory process

Q 53. In diabetic ketoacidosis

A. Treatment corrects hyperglycaemia more quickly than ketoacidosis

B. A large sodium deficit exists

C. Typical anion gap is 13–17 mmol/L

D. Total body potassium is increased

E. Ketonuria accounts for a large part of the osmotic diuresis that is seen

Q 54. Fat embolism syndrome is associated with

A. Renal transplant

B. Systemic lupus erythematosus

C. Animal bites

D. Sickle cell disease

E. Enteral feeding

Q 55. In the APACHE II scoring system

A. There are 34 physiological variables

B. Scores are weighted for age

C. Scores are weighted for chronic disease

D. The system can be used to predict individual patient outcomes

E. A revised Glasgow coma score is incorporated

Q 56. Factors associated with increased mortality in patients with community-acquired pneumonia include

A. Male sex

B. Staphylococcal infection

C. Glucose <5 mmol/L

D. Sodium <130 mmol/L

E. Urea >7 mmol/L

Q 57. *E.coli* 0157

A. Is a common gut commensal

B. Causes haemolytic uraemic syndrome

C. Case reports have fallen in number during the past 20 years
D. Is the commonest cause of acute renal failure in children
E. May be treated by adjunct verocytotoxin therapy

Q 58. Concerning near drowning in children

A. Peripheral vasodilatation characterises the diving reflex
B. Death is frequently due to aspiration of large volumes of liquid into the lungs
C. Serious serum electrolyte abnormalities are common
D. Hypovolaemia is more likely if the child was submersed in salt water than fresh water
E. The chances of survival are inversely related to the rectal temperature on arrival at hospital

Q 59. When assessing the Glasgow Coma Score (GCS)

A. A flexion response to a painful stimulus is always abnormal
B. An extension response to a painful stimulus is sometimes abnormal
C. The more abnormal response to a painful stimulus should be recorded when the responses of two different limbs differ
D. The result is only applicable to patients who have sustained a head injury
E. Firm pressure applied over the patient's sternum constitutes an appropriate painful stimulus

Q 60. Concerning carbon monoxide poisoning

A. The half-life of COHb is 250 min when breathing air and 50 min breathing 100% oxygen
B. Bicarbonate therapy is indicated
C. Dantrolene is of benefit
D. Cherry-red appearance is more common than cyanosis
E. COHb causes pulse oximetry to tend towards 85%

Q 1. For a rapid sequence induction

- **A.** Cricoid pressure should be applied in line with the fourth cervical vertebral body
- **B.** A nasogastric tube should be removed
- **C.** A suction unit capable of generating at least −200 kPa should be immediately available
- **D.** The BURP manoeuvre helps prevent a rise in intragastric pressure
- **E.** Cricoid pressure should be released if a laryngeal mask airway (LMA) needs to be inserted

Q 2. Laryngeal mask airways may be sterilised by

- **A.** Autoclave
- **B.** γ-irradiation
- **C.** Chlorhexidine immersion
- **D.** Ethylene oxide
- **E.** Ultrasonic cleansing

Q 3. Postdural puncture headache

- **A.** Occurs in over 80% cases following puncture of the arachnoid mater with a 16 G Tuohy needle
- **B.** Occurs up to 72 h following dural tap
- **C.** Is relieved by epidural blood patch in 90% cases
- **D.** May be associated with neck stiffness in the absence of meningitis
- **E.** Is relieved by abdominal compression

Q 4. The following anaesthetic drugs are prepared as the salts stated

- **A.** Rocuronium bromide
- **B.** Adrenaline hydrochloride
- **C.** Remifentanil citrate

D. Glycopyrronium sulphate

E. Suxamethonium chloride

Q 5. **Soda lime**

A. Is mostly made up of potassium hydroxide

B. Causes decomposition of trichloroethylene

C. Contains 1% calcium hydroxide

D. Causes decomposition of isoflurane

E. Produces heat during its reaction with CO_2

Q 6. **The dibucaine number**

A. Represents the degree of inhibition of plasma cholinesterase by dibucaine

B. Is normally 75–85

C. Is 40–60 in patients with the atypical enzyme

D. Is 15–25 in heterozygotes

E. If the dibucaine number is >70, the paralysis induced by a standard dose of suxamethonium will not be prolonged

Q 7. **Cerebral ischaemia occurring during carotid endarterectomy under general anaesthesia is directly aggravated by**

A. Barbiturates

B. Hypothermia

C. Ketamine

D. Dextran-containing solutions

E. Hypoventilation

Q 8. **Concerning double-lumen endotracheal tubes**

A. A left-sided tube is contraindicated for operations on the left lung

B. A Carlens tube has its endobronchial extension angled to the right

C. Surgical drainage of a postpneumonectomy empyema is an absolute indication

D. The left-sided Robertshaw tube has a ventilation slot in the bronchial cuff

E. The White tube is a right-sided tube

In the recognition and treatment of malignant hyperthermia

    A. Initially there can be tachycardia and hypertension
    B. An average dose of 2.5 mg/kg of dantrolene is required
    C. Suxamethonium increases jaw muscle tone in all patients
    D. Treatment includes dantrolene with a calcium channel blocker
    E. Doses of neuromuscular-blocking agents should be reduced when dantrolene is used

Q 10. **In a patient presenting for renal transplantation**

    A. Suxamethonium is contraindicated
    B. Blood transfusion is unlikely to be of benefit
    C. Vecuronium elimination is impaired post-transplantation
    D. Systemic infection is a contraindication to transplantation
    E. Lower extremity ischaemia is induced as part of the operative procedure

Q 11. **Day case surgery is appropriate for**

    A. Operations lasting up to 3 h
    B. Babies <6 months old
    C. Patients on whom epidurals are performed
    D. Accompanied patients who do not have a telephone
    E. ASA II patients

Q 12. **Concerning Magnetic Resonance Imaging (MRI)**

    A. Modern cerebral vascular aneurysm clips are MRI compatible
    B. The anaesthetist must leave the scanner when the scan is in progress
    C. MRI scanning is contraindicated if the patient has an artificial pacemaker
    D. Precautions need not be taken while the scan is not in progress
    E. Only nuclei with an odd number of protons or neutrons respond to the magnetic resonance

Q13. **Complications of blood transfusion include**

    A. A rise in body temperature
    B. Appearance of hives on the patient

Exam 3

Questions

C. Appearance of red urine
D. Haemolytic reactions despite giving compatible cross-matched blood
E. Pain

Q 14. Complications of retrobulbar blockade for cataract surgery include

A. Bradycardia
B. Retinal detachment
C. Brain stem anaesthesia
D. Vitreous haemorrhage
E. Optic nerve damage

Q 15. Recovery rooms

A. The first dedicated recovery rooms were opened in the UK
B. Should have 1.5 bays per operating theatre
C. Should be staffed at a ratio of 0.5 nurses per acute bay
D. Were introduced into the USA in 1955
E. Were first described by Florence Nightingale

Q 16. During brachial plexus blockade

A. The interscalene approach commonly leads to inadequate blockade of the ulnar nerve
B. The axillary approach may lead to Horner's syndrome
C. The supraclavicular approach commonly leads to inadequate blockade of the axillary nerve
D. Bilateral interscalene blocks should be used for bilateral shoulder manipulation surgery
E. The axillary approach commonly leads to inadequate blockade of the median nerve

Q 17. Factors predisposing to opioid-related bradycardia include

A. The use of calcium channel blockers
B. Laryngoscopy
C. The presence of β-blockade
D. Rapid IV administration of the opioid
E. Use of suxamethonium

Q 18. **Rocuronium**

    A. Causes a tachycardia

    B. Is physically incompatible with thiopentone

    C. Has two known active metabolites

    D. Is 30% excreted in urine

    E. ED90 is 0.3 mg/kg

Q 19. **Compound A**

    A. Is a metabolite of sevoflurane and trichloroethylene

    B. Is also known as fluoromethyl-2,2-difluoro-1-(trifluoromethyl) vinyl ether

    C. Production is lessened by cooling the soda lime

    D. Contraindicates the use of sevoflurane at fresh gas flows $<2,000$ ml

    E. Production is greater in the presence of baralyme than soda lime

Q 20. **Xenon**

    A. Is non-explosive, colourless and odourless

    B. Has a MAC greater than nitrous oxide

    C. Is a moderate cardiovascular depressant

    D. Is a very dense gas

    E. Has a blood/gas coefficient that is less than that of nitrous oxide

Q 21. **Concerning myocardial contractility**

    A. Measuring myocardial contractility requires that 'preload', 'afterload' and heart rate are constant

    B. The first derivative of the arterial pressure has been used as a measure of myocardial contractility

    C. In the isolated heart, ratio of left ventricular end systolic pressure and volume is a preload independent measure of contractility

    D. In the normal heart agents that increase contractility decrease lusitropy

    E. Dopexamine has no β_1 activity and does not increase myocardial contractility

Exam 3

Questions

Q 22. Concerning nitric oxide

A. Nitric oxide is synthesised from L-arginine in endothelial cells

B. Nitric oxide mediates vascular smooth muscle relaxation via cyclic adenosine monophosphate

C. Nitric oxide powerfully relaxes bronchial smooth muscle

D. Systemically absorbed nitric oxide is metabolised to nitrate with the formation of methaemoglobin

E. Inhaled nitric oxide is supplied from cylinders premixed with an appropriate concentration of oxygen

Q 23. In the stomach

A. Parietal cells are mainly situated around the pylorus

B. Chief cells secrete gastrin

C. Pepsinogen and HCl are secreted by the parietal cells

D. Pepsinogen secretion is increased by vagal stimulation

E. Gastric distension leads to increased acid secretion

Q 24. Concerning the lungs

A. Type 1 alveolar epithelial cells are particularly sensitive to damage from high concentrations of oxygen

B. Pulmonary vascular resistance can be measured in $dynes \cdot sec \cdot cm^{-5}$

C. In an awake subject in the left lateral position, ventilation is greatest in the upper lung

D. In an anaesthetised and paralysed subject in the left lateral position, ventilation is greatest in the upper lung

E. In an anaesthetised subject in the left lateral position, blood flow is greatest in the lower lung

Q 25. Concerning pain

A. Hyperalgesia is an increased response to a stimulus that is normally painful

B. Hyperalgesia develops in normal people after cutaneous injury

C. Allodynia is pain due to a stimulus that does not normally evoke pain

D. Both A delta and C fibres are connected to nociceptors consisting of free nerve endings

E. Both A delta and C fibre nociceptors progressively increase their excitation threshold in response to repeated noxious stimuli

Q 26. Radiofrequency ablation

A. Uses a heated probe to produce a lesion

B. Induces a target temperature of typically 45°C

C. Producing a small lesion requires current flow to a small secondary electrode

D. Lesions are usually conical and are formed 5 mm from the probe tip

E. Requires homogeneous tissue to produce a reliable lesion

Q 27. Concerning acute myocardial infarction (MI)

A. WHO diagnosis on ECG requires >1 mm ST elevation in the standard leads

B. ST elevation in the ECG and history suggestive of acute MI will be supported by angiographic evidence in >90% of cases

C. Thrombolysis re-establishes early coronary flow (equivalent to unaffected arteries) in more than 75% of cases

D. Renal failure is a significant risk factor for cardiovascular death after elective general anaesthesia

E. 6 months after a successfully thrombolysed MI approximately one third of coronary arteries will have re-occluded

Q 28. Concerning myasthenia gravis (MG)

A. Pregnancy may precipitate weakness

B. A preoperative short course of high-dose corticosteroids is used to optimise patients

C. There is a potentiated response to tetanic stimulation

D. Patients presenting for thymectomy can expect their MG to improve in the postoperative period

E. Patients taking in excess of 750 mg of pyridostigmine orally per day are at increased risk of requiring postoperative ventilation

Q 29. In Duchenne muscular dystrophy

A. Muscle innervation is impaired
B. Inheritance is autosomal recessive
C. Proximal muscles are particularly affected
D. Death generally occurs between the ages of 40 and 50 years
E. Pneumonia is the commonest cause of death

Q 30. Myasthenic syndrome

A. Complicates about 10% of bronchogenic carcinomas
B. More commonly affects females
C. Commonly involves bulbar muscles
D. Symptoms are improved by anticholinesterases
E. Produces resistance to suxamethonium

Q 31. Cystic fibrosis

A. Causes sweat to have an abnormally low sodium concentration
B. Is autosomal recessive
C. Causes respiratory secretions to have an abnormally low chloride concentration
D. Is associated with nasal polyps
E. Is associated with intestinal obstruction

Q 32. Acute liver failure

A. Causes hypertension due to encephalopathy
B. Is more commonly associated in the UK with an infective cause rather than hepatotoxins
C. Is complicated by cerebral oedema in 80% cases
D. Is commonly associated with oliguric renal failure
E. From paracetamol overdose occurs as a result of glutathione depletion

Q 33. Rheumatoid arthritis

A. Causes atlantoaxial subluxation in approximately 25% of cases
B. Is associated with an obstructive respiratory defect
C. Is associated with a restrictive respiratory defect

D. Causing more than 4 mm between the odontoid peg and arch of the atlas is associated with cord compression

E. Causes constrictive pericarditis with an annual incidence of approximately 0.4%

Q 34. Concerning patients with pre-eclampsia

A. The commonest cause of maternal death in pre-eclampsia is intracranial haemorrhage

B. An abnormal clotting screen occurs in 50% of patients with a normal platelet count

C. There is a good correlation between central venous pressure and pulmonary artery occlusion pressure in severe pre-eclampsia

D. Magnesium sulphate prior to induction can successfully reduce the pressor response to intubation

E. Angiotensin converting enzyme inhibitors (ACEIs) can be used at term to control blood pressure

Q 35. In patients with cardiac disease undergoing non-cardiac surgery

A. There is strong correlation between the location of a myocardial infarct and the site and severity of coronary artery lesions

B. There should be an 8-hour 'patch free' interval for patients prescribed GTN patches for more than 24 h

C. Patients prescribed ACE inhibitors for LVF are at significant risk of hypotension on induction

D. Non-insulin-dependent diabetics with perioperative myocardial infarction will benefit from tight glucose control with insulin

E. The threshold for advising coronary artery surgery before another operation is lower than for advising coronary artery surgery alone

Q 36. Patients following heart-lung transplantation

A. Usually have a good cough reflex

B. Pleural biopsy is the best procedure for investigating if rejection is occurring

C. Resting heart rate is normal, but there is little change with stimulation
D. Coronary blood flow is generally poor
E. There is an increased incidence of pancreatitis following surgery

Q 37. In orthopaedic surgery

A. Arthroscopy of the knee can be performed under local infiltration anaesthesia
B. Scoliosis surgery is now associated with minimal blood loss
C. Bone cement implantation syndrome is potentiated by intravascular volume deficit
D. Cervical fusion surgery may be done via an anterior or a posterior approach
E. Blood loss during hip surgery is less with general than with regional anaesthesia

Q 38. These conditions present with loss of weight, anaemia, and slight lemon yellow skin appearance

A. Carcinoma of the stomach
B. Carcinoma of the caecum
C. Autoimmune thyroiditis
D. Pernicious anaemia
E. Uraemia

Q 39. Concerning local anaesthesia for intraocular surgery

A. General anaesthesia is more frequently used than local anaesthesia
B. The eyelid is held open by orbicularis oculi
C. The oculocardiac reflex is prevented by insertion of a regional block
D. An axial length of >26 mm indicates a large eye
E. Amaurosis is a common feature of peribulbar injections of local anaesthetic

Q 40. Concerning the pancreas

A. Somatostatin is secreted by the D cells and inhibits secretion of insulin, glucagon and pancreatic polypeptide

B. Applying the Ranson criteria to diagnose pancreatitis requires the measurement of amylase

C. CT scanning in patients with pancreatitis provides prognostic information

D. Ampicillin is an appropriate antibiotic to treat pancreatic infection

E. Early surgical intervention in pancreatitis is contraindicated

Q 41. Concerning pulse oximetry

A. Recordings are accurate to saturations of 30%

B. In the presence of methaemoglobin, measured saturation tends towards 85%

C. Severe tricuspid incompetence may lead to falsely low readings

D. Administration of intravenous methylene blue gives a falsely high reading

E. The presence of deep jaundice may lead to inaccurate readings

Q 42. Concerning capnometry

A. Carbon dioxide in the expired gas after intubation confirms that the tube is correctly placed in the trachea

B. It may help detect circulatory failure

C. Any compound A present is registered as carbon dioxide

D. Mainstream analysers may contribute to 'disconnect' incidents

E. Sidestream analysers cause a 'leak' in the circuit

Q 43. Concerning respiratory function tests

A. The forced expiratory volume in 1s (FEV_1) to forced vital capacity (FVC) ratio is reduced in restrictive lung disease

B. The forced vital capacity (FVC) may be reduced in both restrictive and obstructive lung disease

C. The maximum expiratory flow-volume curve allows differentiation between obstruction in small and large airways

D. Peak expiratory flow rate is sex dependent

E. Forced vital capacity is reduced by approximately 50% following major abdominal surgery

Q 44. Transoesophageal echocardiography (TOE)

A. Can estimate end-systolic and end-diastolic ventricular volumes

B. Can measure ejection fraction

C. With colour flow imaging demonstrates valvular dysfunction

D. Detects myocardial ischaemia by demonstrating regional wall motion abnormalities

E. Is a useful diagnostic technique for detecting dissecting thoracic aortic aneurysms

Q 45. Regarding gas flow measurement

A. The Bourdon gauge is a fixed orifice device

B. The Benedict Roth spirometer involves a bell and rotating drum

C. The vitalograph has a motor-driven chart and bellows

D. A dry gas meter is better for measuring small volumes

E. The vitalograph is not very portable

Q 46. Regarding humidification

A. The water bath method is inefficient because of the large bubble size

B. Latent heat of vaporisation reduces efficiency of the hot rod humidifier

C. Hot element humidifiers are suitable for use with volatile agents

D. Droplets produced by nebulisers may form pools of water if over 5 μ

E. Larger nebulised droplets are a source of cross infection

Q 47. In circulatory shock

A. A raised central venous pressure (CVP) can be used to distinguish between hypovolaemia and septic shock

B. A raised systemic vascular resistance (SVR) will help distinguish between hypovolaemia and cardiogenic shock

C. Cardiac output is raised in hypovolaemic shock

D. Shock may be present without hypotension

E. Nitric oxide synthetase inhibitors have a role in hypovolaemic shock

Q 48. Concerning inotropes

A. The α-adrenergic effects are mediated through a cyclic AMP pathway
B. All inotropes increase intracellular calcium ion levels
C. Dopexamine is an ino-constrictor
D. The potential for digoxin toxicity is increased in hypermagnesaemia
E. Phosphodiesterase inhibitors should not be used in patients with severe heart failure

Q 49. Magnesium in the treatment of acute severe asthma

A. Is an appropriate first-line therapy
B. Should be given as a single dose of 8 mmol
C. May be given to children over 5 years of age
D. Causes clinically significant hypotension
E. Inhibits acetylcholine release at the neuromuscular junction

Q 50. Regarding anaphylaxis

A. It occurs following 'classical pathway' complement activation
B. Bronchospasm is the most common physical sign
C. Elevation of C3 and C4 complement level indicates 'alternative pathway' activation
D. Methylhistamine is measurable in the urine up to 3 h following a reaction
E. Mast cell tryptase is measurable in the blood up to 3 h following a reaction

Q 51. The following drugs may be used in the treatment of status epilepticus

A. Diazepam
B. Thiopentone
C. Sodium valproate
D. Lamotrigene
E. Phenytoin

Q 52. Hyperosmolar non-ketotic coma

A. Is less common than ketoacidosis
B. Usually occurs in a previously undiagnosed diabetic

C. May be precipitated by antibiotic administration
D. Is associated with a mortality of 50%
E. Causes impairment of consciousness which is directly related to serum osmolality

Q 53. Nephrogenic diabetes insipidus

A. Is caused by a deficiency of antidiuretic hormone
B. Is seen after severe head injury
C. May be caused by frusemide administration
D. May be caused by glibenclamide administration
E. May be seen in hyperkalaemia

Q 54. In fat embolism syndrome

A. Presentation usually occurs in the first 24 h following the initial insult
B. The classic syndrome involves pulmonary, cutaneous and renal manifestations
C. The petechial rash is commonly found on the dependent parts of the body
D. Headache and irritability occasionally occur
E. Fat in the urine is a useful diagnostic finding

Q 55. The Glasgow coma scale

A. Scores 1 to 4 for verbal response
B. Has a paediatric version that must be used for small children
C. Was developed for use in medical coma patients
D. Score of 9 represents coma
E. Defines five levels of possible outcome

Q 56. The following serological markers are found in the blood during acute infection with the hepatitis B virus (HBV)

A. Anti-HBs antibody
B. Anti-HBe antibody
C. HBs antigen
D. HBe antigen
E. Anti-HBc (IgM) antibody

Q 57. *E.coli* 0157 infection

    A. Is possible from contact with sheep
    B. Is more common in younger livestock
    C. Is associated with a mortality >50%
    D. Is associated with children's paddling pools
    E. Causes thrombotic thrombocytopaenic purpura in adults

Q 58. Following salicylate overdose

    A. Hypokalaemia is common
    B. Pulmonary oedema occurs in the presence of hypovolaemia
    C. Oxidative phosphorylation is stimulated
    D. Urinary pH is initially alkaline
    E. Forced acid diuresis increases salicylate excretion

Q 59. Following a severe thermal injury

    A. Sepsis is the leading cause of death
    B. Cellular immunity is enhanced
    C. Ambient temperature should be kept below 25°C to minimise the increase in core temperature
    D. An early permeability defect occurs in the lungs regardless of the presence or absence of an associated inhalation injury
    E. The barrier function of the gut to infecting organisms is immediately compromised

Q 60. Hypothermia leads to

    A. Reduced insulin secretion
    B. Prolongation of the PR interval
    C. No cerebral activity at 18°C
    D. Unconsciousness at 34°C
    E. Ventricular fibrillation at 32°C

Q 1. Parathyroid surgery

A. Should not be undertaken if plasma calcium is above 2.6 mmol/L

B. Hyperparathyroidism and phaeochromocytoma co-exist in patients with the multiple endocrine neoplasia syndrome

C. The ECG shows a prolonged Q-T interval with hypercalcaemia

D. Hyperventilation will lower serum ionised calcium levels

E. Hypercalcaemia causes reversible impairment of renal concentrating ability

Q 2. Effects of epidural blockade include

A. A greater degree of hypotension when adrenaline-containing local anaesthetics are used

B. Sympathetic blockade before sensory blockade

C. Anterior spinal artery syndrome

D. Reduced tidal volume with a normal block to T4

E. Reduced peristalsis

Q 3. Concerning gas cylinders

A. Nitrous oxide cylinders are pressurised to 137 bar

B. Carbon dioxide cylinders contain liquid CO_2

C. A size E oxygen cylinder contains 1,800 L

D. A size E N_2O cylinder contains 680 L

E. The tare weight is the weight of a full cylinder plus valve block

Q 4. The following anaesthetic drugs are prepared as the salts stated

A. Ropivacaine hydrochloride

B. Cisatracurium besylate

C. Ephedrine sulphate

D. Mivacurium chloride

E. Neostigmine butylbromide

Q 5. **The following are true of the circle system**

  A. Fresh gas inflow should enter the circuit between the expiratory valve and the patient

  B. It is most efficient when the unidirectional valves are close to the patient

  C. Rebreathing can occur if the directional valves stick closed

  D. Sevoflurane is degraded in soda lime

  E. Phenolphthalein turns white when the absorbent is exhausted

Q 6. **The following have been identified as independent risk factors for perioperative cardiac morbidity**

  A. Hypertension

  B. Diabetes mellitus

  C. Stable angina pectoris

  D. Congestive cardiac failure

  E. Dysrhythmias

Q 7. **The following drugs should be omitted on the day of surgery in a patient who is to undergo TURP under general anaesthesia**

  A. Amiodarone

  B. Aspirin

  C. Atenolol

  D. Chlorthalidone

  E. Enalapril

Q 8. **During one-lung anaesthesia**

  A. Hypercapnia is common

  B. Hypoxaemia is less severe if the collapsed lung is normal

  C. Positive end-expiratory pressure (PEEP) to the dependent lung is contraindicated

  D. Inhalational anaesthetic agents impair hypoxic pulmonary vasoconstriction

  E. True anatomical shunt is partially corrected by increasing the inspired oxygen concentration (FiO_2)

Q 9. During dental surgery

A. Arrhythmias are common during general anaesthesia
B. The Jorgensen technique is a recognised sedation method
C. The Goldman mask can be employed
D. The McKesson mask provides a more reliable oral airway than a conventional facemask
E. Cardiovascular collapse can occur with dental nerve blocks

Q 10. During laser surgery to the airway

A. Theatre personnel should wear goggles to prevent retinal damage from ultraviolet radiation
B. Reduction of FiO_2 with nitrous oxide helps prevent airway fire
C. The laser beam can penetrate a metal endotracheal tube
D. The endotracheal tube should be removed in the event of an airway fire
E. Nd:YAG lasers are more destructive than CO_2 lasers

Q 11. The following are true

A. The left-handed laryngoscope developed by Penlon is for use by left-handed anaesthetists
B. When sterilising anaesthetic equipment, boiling is suitable for those items made from rubber
C. When using the oxygen flush of an anaesthetic machine, the fresh gas flow and volatiles become diluted with oxygen
D. The British standard taper for tracheal tube adaptors is 22 mm
E. Passive scavenging systems have a water trap

Q 12. When considering carotid endarterectomy

A. Regional anaesthesia has been shown to reduce the incidence of postoperative stroke
B. Postoperative TIAs are most likely to be due to microemboli
C. Seizures are a complication of regional anaesthesia
D. Stump pressures reflect adequacy of cerebral perfusion
E. Bilateral endarterectomy causes loss of carotid body function

Q 13. Phaeochromocytoma surgery

A. Preoperatively β-blockers are the first line of treatment
B. Patients may have catecholamine-induced myocarditis
C. The half-life of plasma catecholamines is approximately 45 s
D. Untreated patients suffer from chronic hypovolaemia
E. α-blockers can cause nasal stuffiness

Q 14. Laparoscopic surgery is associated with

A. Right main bronchus intubation
B. A decrease in cardiac output, but only if the patient is supine and horizontal or head up
C. Pneumothorax
D. An increase in arterial carbon dioxide tension if nitrous oxide is the insufflating gas
E. Compartment syndrome

Q 15. Published recommendations for the safe conduct of obstetric anaesthesia in the UK state

A. That the anaesthetist must under no circumstances leave his/her patient
B. Consent for any procedure must be written
C. Patients undergoing regional anaesthetic techniques should spend at least 30 min in recovery
D. All obstetric units should have at least 4 units of uncrossmatched O negative blood
E. The time from informing the anaesthetist to the start of emergency operative delivery should not exceed 15 min

Q 16. Anatomical variations associated with difficult intubation include

A. An increased posterior depth of the mandible
B. A reduced anterior depth of the mandible
C. An absent atlanto-axial gap
D. An increased atlanto-occipital gap
E. A thyromental distance <6 cm

Q 17. Context-sensitive half-time is

A. Dependent upon duration of the infusion
B. Dependent upon excretion
C. Longer for fentanyl than for alfentanil after an infusion lasting 1 h
D. Constant for remifentanil
E. Shorter if the duration of the infusion is long and the apparent volume of distribution at steady state is large rather than small

Q 18. With regard to vitamins

A. A is water soluble
B. Thiamine deficiency can cause heart failure
C. B12 deficiency causes defective DNA synthesis
D. B1 deficiency leads to Wernicke-Korsakoff syndrome
E. Cholecalciferol is 25-hydroxylated in the kidney

Q 19. Ketamine

A. Is metabolised in the liver to an active metabolite
B. Is an imidazole derivative
C. Emergence phenomena may be reduced by co-administration of benzodiazepines and opioids
D. Bronchoconstriction may occur
E. Recovery is rapid via redistribution

Q 20. Thiopentone

A. Is 80% protein bound
B. Follows first-order kinetics which may become zero order at higher doses
C. Is given rectally as a 5 or 10% solution
D. If injected intra-arterially should be followed by hyaluronidase
E. Causes a tachycardia due to a decrease in vagal tone

Q 21. Hypocapnia may cause

A. Increased placental blood flow
B. Hypercalcaemia

C. Hypokalaemia
   D. Reduced cerebral blood flow
   E. Confusion

Q 22. Concerning the splanchnic circulation

   A. The adult liver normally receives approximately 1/3 of its blood supply from the coeliac axis
   B. β_1-adrenergic receptors cause mesenteric arteriolar vasodilatation
   C. Positive end-expiratory pressure (PEEP) decreases portal blood flow
   D. Arcades of arterioles supplying mucosal villi terminate and branch at the tip supplying well-oxygenated blood to the mucosa
   E. The splanchnic venous system can contain 1/3 of the total blood volume

Q 23. Absorption

   A. Of fat occurs after breakdown into monoglycerides
   B. Of bile salts occurs in the jejunum
   C. Of carbohydrate is mainly by active transport
   D. Of iron is in the ileum
   E. Of B_{12} is in the terminal ileum

Q 24. Oxygen

   A. Delivery is approximately 1,000 ml/min
   B. Consumption is approximately 250 ml/min
   C. The lungs store approximately 300 ml after a subject has breathed 100% oxygen
   D. Consumption can be measured by spirometry
   E. $DO_2 = Q \cdot (CaO_2 - CvO_2)$

Q 25. Concerning cellular receptors

   A. Naloxone reverses the analgesia produced by acupuncture
   B. Ketamine acts on the NMDA receptor
   C. Mu opioid receptors stimulate adenylyl cyclase
   D. Histamine receptors are not present in the CNS
   E. Caffeine is an adenosine receptor antagonist

Q 26. Codeine

A. Has an oral bioavailability of approximately 50%
B. Is metabolised by O-demethylation to morphine
C. Cannot be metabolised to morphine by 7% of the Caucasian population
D. Combined paracetamol plus codeine preparations produce an effect indistinguishable from the use of codeine alone
E. Metabolism to morphine is antagonised by tricyclic antidepressants

Q 27. Concerning the heart in an erect PA chest radiogram

A. Kerley 'B' lines are distended pulmonary lymphatic vessels
B. Redistribution of pulmonary vessel size occurs with LA pressures of 16–22 cmH$_2$O
C. The carina forms a border between the aortic knuckle and the left atrial appendage
D. Generally a cardiothoracic ratio >55% is associated with an ejection fraction <40%
E. A 'cottage loaf' shaped cardiac silhouette occurs with total anomalous pulmonary venous drainage

Q 28. Concerning patients with epilepsy

A. The electroencephalogram (EEG) represents the summation of cerebral synaptic activity
B. Carbamazapine is an enzyme inhibitor
C. Rapid intravenous loading of phenytoin causes hypotension
D. Enflurane is used to produce cortical EEG changes for mapping epileptic foci
E. Droperidol and haloperidol should be avoided

Q 29. Hepatitis A

A. Is the commonest type of viral hepatitis
B. Spread is usually faecal-oral
C. Has an incubation time of approximately 6 months
D. Can lead to a chronic carrier state
E. Has an acute mortality of approximately 10%

Q 30. **Dystrophia myotonica**

    A. Is associated with cardiomyopathy
    B. Causes decreased suxamethonium sensitivity
    C. Is caused by an abnormality of calcium metabolism
    D. Myotonia is precipitated by cold
    E. Causes delayed gastric emptying due to impaired smooth muscle motility

Q 31. **Sarcoidosis**

    A. Causes lymphopenia
    B. Is commoner in males than females
    C. Typically causes unilateral lymphadenopathy
    D. Is diagnosed using the Kveim test
    E. Can be mimicked by beryllium poisoning

Q 32. **Concerning myasthenia gravis**

    A. Volatile agents lead to a reduction in twitch height
    B. Sensitivity to suxamethonium is increased
    C. All non-depolarising agents lead to an increased degree of neuromuscular block
    D. The presence of circulating anti-acetylcholine receptor antibodies is a reliable diagnostic sign
    E. Anticholinesterase therapy should be recommenced 48 h after surgery

Q 33. **Haemophilia A**

    A. The gene for haemophilia is located on chromosome 7
    B. Is associated with a prolonged bleeding time
    C. 50% of haemophilia carriers warrant haematological prophylaxis prior to major surgery
    D. Deamino-D-arginine vasopressin can provide prophylaxis in mild haemophilia for major surgery
    E. Factor VIII usually has a half-life of 12 h

Q 34. **Regarding thromboembolism in pregnancy**

    A. Pulmonary thromboembolism is the commonest cause of maternal death in the UK
    B. The incidence of fatal pulmonary thromboembolism has been increasing over the last decade

C. Approximately 90% of deep vein thrombosis affects the left side in pregnancy

D. The activated partial thromboplastin time is an unreliable monitor of heparin activity in pregnancy

E. Ventilation-perfusion scanning is contraindicated in pregnancy

Q 35. In ENT and maxillo-facial surgery

A. A Le Fort I fracture involves the nose

B. A Le Fort III fracture results in the complete separation of the maxillary complex from the skull

C. Changing the endotracheal tube is necessary during laryngectomy

D. The mortality for children requiring re-operation for bleeding following tonsillectomy and adenoidectomy is approximately 1 in 500

E. Epiglottitis is usually caused by *H. Influenzae* type B

Q 36. In gastrointestinal surgery

A. A Hartmann's procedure involves bowel resection and re-anastomosis

B. An anterior resection is the operation of choice for carcinomas of the lower third of the rectum

C. A three-stage oesophagectomy usually involves an incision on the left side of the neck

D. A pharyngeal pouch most commonly occurs between the inferior constrictor of the pharynx and cricopharyngeus

E. Barrett's oesophagus occurs due to persistent gastro-oesophageal reflux

Q 37. In obstetrics

A. Tocolysis may be produced with β-2 adrenoceptor agonists

B. Therapeutic serum levels of magnesium are 4–6 mg/L

C. Glyceryl trinitrate may be used intravenously to obtain uterine relaxation

D. A foetus in the occiput posterior position will require Caesarean section

E. The death rate associated with Caesarean section is approximately 1 in 2,000

Q 38. Concerning anaesthesia for thyroid surgery

- **A.** The skin over the thyroid is supplied by the brachial plexus
- **B.** Regional anaesthesia may impair respiratory function
- **C.** Laryngospasm occurring 24 h postoperatively is likely to be due to nerve irritation
- **D.** The majority of retrosternal goitres require a sternal incision
- **E.** Thyroid carcinoma is associated with phaeochromocytoma

Q 39. Indications to proceed to surgery in necrotising enterocolitis include

- **A.** Pneumoperitoneum
- **B.** Intestinal gangrene
- **C.** Intestinal obstruction
- **D.** Gastrointestinal haemorrhage
- **E.** Abdominal tenderness

Q 40. The stress response to surgery involves the following changes

- **A.** Increased thyroid stimulating hormone (TSH) secretion
- **B.** Decreased insulin secretion
- **C.** Increased renin secretion
- **D.** Increased aldosterone secretion
- **E.** Increased testosterone secretion

Q 41. Concerning the electrocardiogram (ECG)

- **A.** It provides continuous monitoring of the circulation
- **B.** Standard lead II is the best monitor of anterior descending coronary artery territory
- **C.** It provides a highly sensitive monitor of myocardial ischaemia
- **D.** CM5 monitoring requires the left arm electrode to be placed in the left anterior axillary line in the 5th intercostal space
- **E.** Leads V4–V6 monitor the circumflex artery territory

Q 42. When measuring gas flows

- **A.** The Wright's respirometer is an anemometer
- **B.** The Datex Ultima monitor utilises a vane flow meter
- **C.** The Wright's respirometer measures flow in both directions

D. Flow can be measured using thermistors

E. Flow can be measured using ultrasound

Q 43. Regarding the gas laws

A. Charles's law states that at constant pressure the volume of a given mass of gas varies directly with the absolute temperature

B. The third gas law states that at constant temperature volume varies inversely with pressure

C. Adiabatic changes are those that involve changes in the state of a gas without transfer of heat with the surroundings

D. Dalton's law states that equal volumes of gases at the same temperature and pressure contain equal numbers of molecules

E. 101.3 kPa is equal to 750 mmHg

Q 44. At high altitudes

A. A variable-bypass vaporiser will deliver the set concentration

B. A TEC 6 vaporiser will deliver the set concentration

C. A variable-bypass vaporiser will deliver the same partial pressure as at sea level

D. A TEC 6 vaporiser will deliver the same partial pressure as at sea level

E. MAC remains unaffected

Q 45. The following tests indicate inadequate or partial reversal of neuromuscular blockade

A. A head lift sustained for 3 seconds

B. A maximum inspiratory pressure of $-20\,cmH_2O$

C. Lack of handgrip

D. A post-tetanic count of 8

E. An arterial $PCO_2 > 6.5\,kPa$

Q 46. The fuel cell

A. Utilises a platinum cathode

B. Current flow depends on uptake of oxygen at the anode

C. Commonly incorporates potassium chloride as the electrolyte

D. Relies on batteries

E. Lifespan depends on the period of time exposed to oxygen

Q 47. The following drugs have cyclic-AMP-dependent positive inotropic effects at clinical doses

A. Digoxin
B. Glucagon
C. Calcium salts
D. Thyroxine
E. Aminophylline

Q 48. The following are accepted diagnostic criteria for acute respiratory distress Syndrome (ARDS)

A. Unilateral diffuse pulmonary infiltrates on the chest X-ray
B. Partial pressure (kPa) to inspired oxygen ratio (PaO_2/FiO_2) <20, despite a normal $PaCO_2$
C. Pulmonary capillary wedge pressure (PCWP) >20 mmHg
D. Known triggering event or risk factor
E. Pulmonary infection

Q 49. When establishing whether brain stem death has occurred

A. Doll's eye movements should be present
B. Hypothermia must be corrected to at least 36°C
C. The cause of the coma must be established
D. More than 6 h should have elapsed since the event that caused the suspected brain stem death
E. The presence of plantar reflexes excludes the diagnosis

Q 50. Regarding human immunodeficiency virus (HIV) infection

A. Serum which does not contain anti-HIV antibodies may be positive for p24 antigen
B. Initial infection by HIV-1 is associated with an acute seroconversion illness in 60% of patients
C. The presence of pneumocystis carinii pneumonia (PCP) distinguishes HIV from other immunodeficiency disorders
D. PCP is characteristically associated with fever and a productive cough
E. Infection with cryptococcus neoformans usually presents as intractable secretory diarrhoea

Q 51. The following cause lactic acidosis

- **A.** Bartter's syndrome
- **B.** Metformin
- **C.** Thiamine deficiency
- **D.** Corticosteroids
- **E.** Anaemia

Q 52. Regarding burns

- **A.** The presence of a significant inhalational injury is associated with a 10% mortality
- **B.** Suxamethonium should be avoided in any patient with >25% burns
- **C.** Carbon monoxide has an affinity for haemoglobin 4 times that of oxygen
- **D.** Drowsiness occurs at carboxyhaemoglobin levels below 50%
- **E.** Mortality in patients with major burns has remained essentially unchanged for the last 50 years

Q 53. Regarding Guillian Barre syndrome

- **A.** It may be purely sensory
- **B.** Approximately a third of patients require ventilatory support
- **C.** If associated with preceding *Campylobacter jejuni* enteritis, it carries a worse prognosis
- **D.** Antibodies to *Campylobacter jejuni* occur more commonly in patients with the axonal form of the disease
- **E.** CSF opening pressure at lumbar puncture is typically elevated

Q 54. The following are associated with acute pancreatitis

- **A.** Metronidazole
- **B.** Campylobacter infection
- **C.** Duodenal ulceration
- **D.** Systemic lupus erythematosus
- **E.** Pregnancy

Q 55. Regarding nutrition in renal failure

- **A.** Endogenous urea can be converted to amino acids
- **B.** A high carbohydrate load is considered beneficial

C. Low osmolality feeds are better tolerated
D. A high-protein diet is required
E. Amino acids can be administered via dialysate solutions

Q 56. Pacemakers

A. The first letter of the pacemaker code relates to the chamber sensed
B. May be unipolar or bipolar
C. Can be re-programmed by diathermy
D. May be inhibited by suxamethonium
E. A threshold value of 10 V for a temporary pacemaker is normal

Q 57. During an asthma attack

A. A normal $PaCO_2$ is a good prognostic marker
B. There is flow-dependent collapse of the small airways
C. The transfer factor for carbon monoxide may increase
D. Mechanical ventilation with a low inspiratory flow rate increases gas trapping
E. Hypotension during ventilation should be managed with inotropes and fluids

Q 58. High-frequency jet ventilation

A. Causes alveolar gas trapping
B. Does not require the humidification of inspired gases
C. Can only achieve adequate alveolar ventilation if the tidal volume is greater than the anatomical dead space
D. Achieves an increase in alveolar minute ventilation mainly by increasing ventilatory frequency
E. Is suited to the ventilatory management of patients with acute severe asthma

Q 59. Concerning sedation in the Intensive Care Unit

A. The use of alfentanil infusions should be avoided in renal failure
B. Sepsis impairs the metabolism of benzodiazepines
C. Morphine undergoes extrahepatic metabolism

D. The clearance of remifentanil is independent of renal and hepatic function

E. Propofol undergoes minimal metabolism

Q 60. **Concerning the underwater seal used for chest drainage**

A. The drain is likely to be ineffective if the tube volume is >50% of the patient's maximal inspiratory volume

B. The volume of water in the underwater seal must be >50% of the patient's maximal inspiratory volume

C. The end of the tube forming the underwater seal should be >10 cm below the surface of the water for safety

D. A Heimlich valve can be used instead of an underwater seal

E. A fluid trap can be safely placed between the patient and the underwater seal

Q 1. **Concerning pacemakers**

     A. Demand pacemakers cannot be converted to fixed rate
     B. Bipolar diathermy should not be used
     C. Volatile agents do not affect pacemaker activity
     D. A VVI code denotes pacing and sensing of both chambers
     E. Rate-responsive devices can increase pacing rate in response to changes in respiration

Q 2. **The following are anaesthetic implications for a patient with aortic stenosis**

     A. The myocardium is susceptible to ischaemia in the absence of coronary artery disease
     B. The presence of atrial fibrillation is highly significant
     C. Bradycardia induces hypotension
     D. Inotropes should not be used
     E. Left ventricular hypertrophy can be seen electrocardiographically

Q 3. **Enflurane**

     A. Is 2-chloro-1,1,2-trifluoroethyl difluoromethyl ether
     B. Is a yellowish volatile liquid
     C. Is odourless
     D. Has a MAC of 1.68
     E. Causes epileptiform EEG activity

Q 4. **During anaesthesia, cerebral blood flow**

     A. Is 50% supplied by the vertebral arteries
     B. Should normally be 50 ml/100 g/min
     C. To diseased areas may be made worse by hypoventilation
     D. Is increased by suxamethonium administration
     E. Is reduced in a dose-dependent fashion by administration of halothane

Q 5. TURP syndrome

   A. Leads to hypernatraemia
   B. May be ameliorated by giving hypotonic IV infusions
   C. May be avoided by measuring ethanol in the exhaled breath of the patient
   D. Should not occur if the height of the irrigating fluid is limited to 1 m above the patient
   E. Should not occur if the resection time is limited to 120 min

Q 6. During one-lung ventilation

   A. In the lateral position hypoxaemia is due to increased dead space in the upper lung
   B. Hypoxaemia is greatest when there is no pre-existing lung disease
   C. Maintenance of positive end-expiratory pressure to the ventilated lung helps reduce hypoxaemia
   D. Hypoxaemia is generally worst about 10 min after onset of one-lung ventilation
   E. Pulmonary artery ligation of the upper lung can be used to decrease hypoxaemia

Q 7. During neurosurgical anaesthesia the following are regarded as providing an early and sensitive indication of air embolism

   A. Pulmonary artery flotation (Swan-Ganz) catheter
   B. 'Mill-wheel' murmur
   C. Trans-cranial doppler ultrasonography
   D. Capnography
   E. Electrocardiogram

Q 8. The following preoperative findings predict clinically significant pulmonary complications following lung resection

   A. An arterial oxygen tension in air (PaO_2) <9 kPa
   B. An arterial carbon dioxide tension ($PaCO_2$) >6 kPa
   C. A Forced vital capacity (FVC) <70% of the predicted value
   D. A Forced expired volume in 1 s (FEV_1) <1 litre
   E. A maximum breathing capacity (MBC) <50% of the predicted value

Q 9. In pyloric stenosis

A. Hyperchloraemic alkalosis is the characteristic biochemical abnormality
B. The initial renal response is excretion of acid urine
C. Pyloromyotomy should not be delayed if vomiting persists and there is difficulty in correcting the electrolyte abnormalities
D. Normal saline is contraindicated in resuscitation as the neonatal kidney handles salt loads poorly
E. Incomplete correction of the biochemical abnormalities can result in postoperative hyperventilation

Q 10. Post operative nausea and vomiting

A. Is more common if there is a history of motion sickness
B. Is the most common cause of hospital admission following day case surgery
C. Is more likely if laparoscopic procedures are performed at the time of the menses
D. Is reduced in children by preoperative suggestion therapy
E. Occurs in more than 75% children undergoing strabismus surgery without antiemetic cover

Q 11. Soda lime and 'baralyme' differ in the following ways

A. Soda lime contains sodium hydroxide instead of barium hydroxide as the active agent
B. Soda lime does not contain a silica binder
C. Baralyme already contains water
D. Baralyme does not contain calcium hydroxide
E. Soda lime is a more efficient absorber of carbon dioxide

Q 12. In the management of anaesthesia for Jehovah's witnesses

A. A cell saver system is unacceptable
B. A child of 14 cannot legally consent to receive blood
C. Active postoperative cooling can be used as a management strategy
D. Under no circumstances should blood be administered once a consent form has been signed
E. Autotransfusion is unacceptable

Q 13. Consent for anaesthesia and surgery

A. Is valid if verbal
B. The basis of consent is the explanation given to the patient
C. All complications of anaesthesia should be explained
D. Consent should be obtained before the administration of the premedication
E. Written consent is preferable and should be obtained from a relative if the patient is unable to sign

Q 14. The following are recognised complications of positioning

A. Prone : blindness
B. Sitting : intraoral pressure sores
C. Sitting : greater surgical blood loss
D. Lateral : rhabdomyolysis
E. Trendelenburg : lingual nerve neuropathy

Q 15. Concerning the laryngeal mask airway (LMA)

A. A size 1 mask is suitable for patients weighing <5 kg
B. The mask provides protection from aspiration of oropharyngeal blood
C. Insertion of the mask causes a 20% rise in blood pressure
D. The size 5 mask has a bigger internal diameter than a size 10.0 endotracheal tube
E. The size 5 mask has a cuff volume of up to 50 ml

Q 16. The following needles are correctly positioned to perform the stated block

A. Ilioinguinal: 2 cm lateral and caudal to the anterior superior iliac spine
B. Deep cervical plexus: Midway between the mastoid process and greater cornua of the hyoid
C. Sciatic: 3 cm below the midpoint of a line connecting the posterior superior iliac spine with the greater trochanter
D. Median: Between the tendons of palmaris longus and flexor carpi ulnaris at the proximal palmar crease
E. Axillary: Just above the axillary artery as high up in the axilla as possible

Q 17. Opioid-induced muscle rigidity

A. Improves with administration of muscle relaxants
B. Can impair the ability to mechanically ventilate a patient
C. Will usually occur following rapid IV injection of remifentanil 1 μg/kg
D. Is due to a direct opioid action on muscle fibres
E. The duration of action of naloxone exceeds that of remifentanil

Q 18. Rocuronium

A. 0.6 mg/kg provides acceptable intubating conditions within 60 s
B. May trigger malignant hyperthermia (MH)
C. Elimination half-life is unaffected by hepatic disease
D. Duration of action is prolonged by magnesium
E. Has a decreased therapeutic effect in the presence of aminoglycosides

Q 19. Sevoflurane

A. Is a methyl-propyl-ether
B. Has a blood gas solubility of 0.6
C. Has a MAC of 6.0%
D. Is stable in soda lime
E. Is entirely fluorinated

Q 20. Propofol

A. Undergoes a greater degree of protein binding than thiopentone
B. Is licensed for use as an induction agent in infants
C. Has antipruritic properties
D. Reduces cerebral metabolic rate and ICP
E. Is a poorly water-soluble isopropyl phenol

Q 21. Concerning corticosteroids

A. Hydrocortisone is an endogenously produced steroid
B. The normal adult daily cortisol production is 25–30 mg per day
C. The hypothalamic-pituitary axis is suppressed by 5 mg of methylprednisolone per day

D. Addisonian crisis will occur if a patient stops a course of 30 mg per day of prednisolone after 3 weeks of therapy
E. Normal hypothalamic-pituitary-adrenal (HPA) function can be assumed 6 weeks after stopping 'high-dose' corticosteroids

Q 22. At altitude

A. Barometric pressure decreases linearly with altitude
B. Acidic urine would be expected during acclimitisation
C. The oxygen dissociation curve is shifted to the left
D. Pulmonary hypertension occurs
E. Mixed venous blood has a PO_2 of approximately 10 mmHg in long-term residents at 15,000 ft

Q 23. In the kidney

A. Approximately 1,300 ml/min of blood passes through the glomeruli
B. Almost all filtered potassium is reabsorbed in the proximal tubule
C. The juxtaglomerular apparatus secretes angiotensin I
D. Renally produced prostaglandins are mainly vasoconstrictor
E. Insulin catabolism occurs in the kidney

Q 24. Functional residual capacity (FRC)

A. Is the sum of residual volume and expiratory reserve volume
B. Can be measured by helium dilution
C. Is increased in asthma
D. Is increased by anaesthesia with positive pressure ventilation
E. Is normally 1.5–2.0 litres for an average male

Q 25. Acute pain in children

A. A normal 8- year-old child would be expected to be able to use a PCA system
B. The Oucher scale is a method of assessing pain in children
C. At room temperature pure lignocaine and prilocaine are crystalline solids
D. The recommended daily dose of diclofenac for children is 1–3 mg/kg
E. Morphine-6-glucuronide is a more potent mu agonist than morphine

Q 26. Trigeminal neuralgia

A. Is characterised by attacks of intense, lancinating pain lasting about 1 h
B. Commonly interferes with sleep
C. 'Idiopathic' trigeminal neuralgia is sometimes caused by venous compression of the trigeminal nerve roots
D. More than 90% of cases respond well to carbamazapine
E. Is a symptom of multiple sclerosis

Q 27. In peptic ulcer disease

A. Helicobacter pylori is found in between 70 and 90% of patients
B. Gastric hydrochloric acid secretion has a pH of <1
C. Non-steroidal anti-inflammatory drugs are associated with ulcer complications with equal frequency in the stomach and duodenum
D. H2 antagonists are useful prophylaxis against NSAID-induced gastric ulceration
E. Approximately 80% of haemorrhage from peptic ulcers stops spontaneously

Q 28. Concerning patients with atrial fibrillation

A. Aspirin is the drug of choice for preventing stroke in patients over 60
B. Anticoagulation should be continued after successful cardioversion
C. Digoxin reduces the number of attacks in paroxysmal atrial fibrillation
D. Amiodarone induces hepatic enzymes and lowers digoxin levels
E. More than 50% of patients successfully treated with cardioversion relapse in the first year

Q 29. Hepatitis B

A. Is an RNA virus
B. Can be transmitted via saliva
C. Chronic carriage is associated with hepatocellular carcinoma
D. A patient positive for e antigen is highly infectious
E. Infection causes fulminant hepatic failure in approximately 50%

Q 30. Myocarditis can be caused by

- **A.** Rheumatic fever
- **B.** Diabetes mellitus
- **C.** SLE
- **D.** Toxoplasma
- **E.** Coxsackie virus

Q 31. Concerning drug misuse

- **A.** Ecstasy (MDMA) is associated with hyponatraemia
- **B.** Pulmonary oedema may be caused by inhalation of cocaine
- **C.** Ecstasy (MDMA) causes hypothermia
- **D.** Vasopressors reverse the tachydysrhythmic effects of cocaine
- **E.** Cannabis causes tachycardia

Q 32. Sarcoidosis

- **A.** Is a disease characterised by caseating epithelioid granulomas
- **B.** Is a cause of difficult intubation
- **C.** Is a cause of obstructive lung disease
- **D.** Is a cause of complete heart block under general anaesthesia
- **E.** Is a cause of hypercalcaemia

Q 33. Regarding the muscular dystrophies

- **A.** Facioscapulohumeral dystrophy is consistent with a normal lifespan
- **B.** Cardiomyopathy is rare in Duchenne muscular dystrophy
- **C.** There is an increased risk of malignant hyperthermia
- **D.** Duchenne muscular dystrophy is the most common variety
- **E.** Cardiorespiratory impairment is a common anaesthetic concern

Q 34. Concerning heart disease in pregnancy

- **A.** Cardiac output in normal parturients usually increases after delivery of the placenta
- **B.** Cardiovascular disease is the leading non-obstetric cause of maternal death in the UK
- **C.** Pulmonary oedema associated with mitral stenosis should be managed with a β-adrenergic receptor antagonist

D. Pulmonary hypertension is a significant risk factor for postpartum mortality

E. Patients with prosthetic valves are recommended to change to heparin at the beginning and end of pregnancy

Q 35. Concerning patients with phaeochromocytoma

A. 10% of tumours are extra-adrenal

B. Diagnosis involves assaying urinary 5-hydroxyindole acetic acid (HIAA)

C. Are associated with von Recklinghausen's disease

D. Blood glucose should be monitored for 24 h after removal

E. Right-sided tumours are more common and technically more difficult to remove

Q 36. In ophthalmic surgery

A. Normal intraocular pressure is between 10 and 20 mmHg

B. Sulphur hexafluoride is less soluble in water than nitrous oxide

C. Intravitreal gas injected during retinal detachment surgery is usually absorbed within a few hours

D. Myopic eyes usually have a longer axial length than normal eyes

E. Scleral banding for retinal detachment requires the intraocular pressure to be kept low

Q 37. Thyroid surgery

A. May precipitate thyroid storm

B. May precipitate hyperparathyroidism

C. Is considered urgent for thyrotoxic women of child-bearing age who cannot have radioiodine

D. Thyrotoxic patients may need preoperative treatment with β-blockers

E. May result in pneumothorax

Q 38. Concerning neonates with congenital abdominal wall defects

A. Gastroschisis will usually need to be operated on within 24 h

B. Gastroschisis is frequently associated with other congenital anomalies

C. Primary closure of the defect is essential to avoid infection
D. Most neonates can be extubated within 24 h
E. Vaginal delivery is absolutely contraindicated

Q 39. In a patient undergoing TURP

A. Use of normal saline as an irrigant inhibits the cutting properties of the resectoscope
B. Visual disturbance in an awake patient is a sign of TURP syndrome
C. Haemolysis is a common laboratory finding when using glycine as the irrigating fluid in TURP syndrome
D. Hypothermia is less common in patients under general anaesthesia
E. Operative intervention is mandatory when perforation of the bladder is suspected

Q 40. Oesophageal varices

A. Occur with portal hypertension (i.e. portal venous pressure >10 mmHg)
B. May be caused by Budd-Chiari syndrome
C. Treatment with a Sengstaken tube may not require inflation of the oesophageal balloon
D. Intravenous vasopressin or octreotide should be given
E. Glyceryl trinitrate (GTN) infusion may be useful

Q 41. Concerning central venous pressure (CVP) catheter monitoring

A. The CVP may be overestimated in a mechanically ventilated patient if chest wall compliance is low
B. The CVP may be underestimated in a spontaneously ventilating patient if the lung compliance is low
C. The presence of atrial fibrillation produces prominent 'a' waves
D. Tricuspid regurgitation produces cannon 'a' waves
E. Third degree heart block produces giant 'v' waves

Q 42. Regarding oxygen analysis

A. The diamagnetic principle relies on the attraction of oxygen for an electric field
B. Null deflection analysers are very accurate

- **C.** Paramagnetic analysers do not require calibration
- **D.** Paramagnetic molecules have unpaired electrons in the outer shell
- **E.** The fuel cell generates its own battery

Q 43. The following are basic Systeme Internationale (SI) units

- **A.** Candela
- **B.** Kelvin
- **C.** Pascal
- **D.** Hertz
- **E.** Watt

Q 44. The TEC 6 vaporiser

- **A.** Is suitable for sevoflurane
- **B.** Is electrically heated
- **C.** Is pressurised
- **D.** Has two independent gas sources
- **E.** Performs predictably at altitude

Q 45. When measuring gas flow

- **A.** The pneumotachograph provides a continuous measurement of airflow
- **B.** Flow characteristics vary in the pneumotachograph
- **C.** The bubble flowmeter has a variable orifice
- **D.** Temperature changes may affect the calibration of the pneumotachograph
- **E.** The bubble flowmeter is suitable for a wide range of flows

Q 46. The oxygen electrode

- **A.** Relies on a lead anode
- **B.** Cathode is usually platinum
- **C.** Potassium hydroxide commonly forms the electrolyte
- **D.** Current flow depends on oxygen tension at the cathode
- **E.** Cannot be used with blood

Q 47. Thrombolytic therapy

A. Is contraindicated in menstruating patients
B. Is indicated in patients with dominant R waves and ST depression in leads V1–3
C. Is contraindicated in patients with cardiac chest pain of >12 h duration
D. Should be accompanied by heparin therapy
E. Is given by an intravenous single bolus dose regime

Q 48. Recommended management of acute respiratory distress syndrome (ARDS) includes

A. Permissive hypercapnia
B. Extracorporeal membrane oxygenation (ECMO)
C. Early use of corticosteroids
D. Diuretics
E. Mechanical ventilation

Q 49. In severe pancreatitis

A. Calcium replacement should be titrated against total serum calcium
B. Early nasojejunal feeding is recommended
C. Pethidine is the analgesic agent of choice
D. Prophylactic high-dose broad-spectrum antibiotics have been shown to reduce mortality
E. A 3-cm pancreatic pseudocyst should be drained under CT or ultrasound guidance

Q 50. The following pulmonary catheter measurements are compatible with a diagnosis of septic shock

A. Cardiac index = 2.0 L/min/m^2
B. Central venous pressure = 2 mmHg
C. Systemic vascular resistance = 750 dynes $\cdot$ cm $\cdot$ s^{-5}
D. Pulmonary capillary wedge pressure = 19 mmHg
E. Pulmonary vascular resistance = 300 dynes $\cdot$ cm $\cdot$ s^{-5}

Q 51. The following cause a metabolic acidosis with an increased anion gap

A. Trauma
B. Renal tubular acidosis

C. Ureteroenterostomies
D. Hypokalaemia
E. Diarrhoea and vomiting

Q 52. Regarding near drowning

A. Immersion fully dressed into cold water (5°C) drops core temperature by 2°C/h
B. Temperature-related cerebral protection occurs before any significant risk of aspiration and hypoxia
C. Hypothermia is a good prognostic sign in an unconscious drowning victim
D. Early advanced life support is the most important factor in a good outcome
E. Steroids probably improve outcome

Q 53. In acute severe asthma

A. Nitroglycerin has been shown to improve bronchospasm
B. Magnesium reduces bronchoconstriction
C. Aminophylline increases diaphragmatic contractility
D. Bronchodilators may increase V/Q mismatch
E. Helium can be used to reduce the work of breathing

Q 54. Risk factors for pulmonary embolism include

A. Antithrombin III deficiency
B. Anaemia
C. Inflammatory bowel disease
D. Protein S deficiency
E. Electric shock

Q 55. TPN for septic patients

A. Is contraindicated
B. Is ideally formulated as a lipid emulsion
C. Should contain branched-chain amino acids
D. Should have a high glucose content
E. Is an iso-osmotic preparation

Q 56. Urine may be discoloured by

A. Propofol
B. Rifampicin

C. Beetroot

D. L-dopa

E. Porphyria

Q 57. **The following serum tests are invalidated by the presence of high concentrations of IV contrast media**

A. Thyroid function tests

B. Bilirubin

C. Potassium

D. Calcium

E. Clotting studies

Q 58. **Regarding Ranson's criteria to assess the severity of pancreatitis**

A. Evaluations are made on admission and at 24 h

B. The presence of 5 criteria is associated with a mortality of greater than 40%

C. AST above 250 U/L at 24 h is a criterion

D. White cell count above 16,000/mm^3 on admission is a criterion

E. The Imrie score reduces the number of Ranson's criteria without losing predictive power

Q 59. **Acute coronary syndromes**

A. Include non-Q wave myocardial infarction

B. Are initiated by fissuring of an atheromatous plaque

C. Are characterised by stable angina

D. Should ideally be managed in a sitting position

E. Have a worse prognosis if right bundle branch block is identified on the presenting ECG

Q 60. **The following clinical conditions are associated with a prolonged QT interval on the electrocardiogram (ECG)**

A. Hyperparathyroidism

B. Hypothermia

C. Pericarditis

D. Ischaemic heart disease

E. Romano-Ward syndrome

Section 2 – Answers

A 1.   **A.** true   **B.** true   **C.** false   **D.** true   **E.** false

Body mass index (BMI) is defined as weight (kg) divided by height (m) squared. A BMI greater than 28 is regarded as obese. Obese patients metabolise volatiles to a greater extent than others. The blood levels of fluoride after methoxyflurane, halothane and enflurane and the bromide levels after halothane are higher in obesity. It has been implied that fat-soluble volatile agents may have a prolonged elimination time with slower recovery, but clinically for exposures of less than 24 h there is a normal recovery time. Airway maintenance difficulties must be anticipated. Part of the reason is that the laryngeal aperture assumes a more cephalad and anterior position as in small children. Peripheral nerve stimulation is often difficult to assess with a stimulator because of the increased amount of tissue between skin electrode and peripheral nerve. The use of percutaneous needle electrodes has been advocated to circumvent this.

Barash, Cullen, Stoelting. *Clinical Anesthesia*, 2nd Edn. Chapter 42.

A 2.   **A.** false   **B.** false   **C.** true   **D.** false   **E.** true

Lower limb tourniquets are usually inflated to 450–500 mmHg. The use of padding is controversial. If it is used, care should be taken to avoid creases or ridges. If autoclaved, the tourniquet bandage should be allowed to cool adequately before use to reduce the risk of skin damage. There have been several instances where 'burns' have been noted under a tourniquet cuff employed during surgery, some of which required corrective surgery.

Prys-Roberts, Brown. *International Practice of Anaesthesia*. Butterworth Heinemann, Chapter 114.
Safety Notice MDA SN 1999(26)

A 3. **A.** false **B.** false **C.** true **D.** false **E.** true

The Goldman cardiac risk index is a scoring system for preoperative identification of patients at risk from major perioperative cardiovascular complications whilst undergoing non-cardiac surgery. Presence of a third heart sound or an elevated JVP is the highest individual scorer. Other factors include MI within 6 months of procedure, multiple ventricular ectopics, heart rhythm other than sinus, severe aortic stenosis, emergency operation and abdominal or thoracic procedure. Age >70 years is a risk factor. The scoring system has a high sensitivity but a low specificity.

Yentis, Hirsch, Smith. *Anaesthesia A to Z*. Butterworth Heinemann, 1993.

A 4. **A.** true **B.** true **C.** false **D.** true **E.** true

Post dural puncture headaches are due to reduced CSF pressure through leakage via the dural defect. They are classically frontal or occipital, made better when lying flat, and may be accompanied by tinnitus or photophobia. Women are more prone than men. This may be related to the influence of oestrogen and progesterone. It may well be for these reasons that pregnant women have a greater incidence of headache than non-pregnant. Midline approaches to the subarachnoid space result in greater leakage of CSF than paramedian approaches and have a higher headache incidence. Nearly all headaches resolve in time but it is recommended that a blood patch be offered if it does not settle within 24 h with hydration, analgesics and bed rest.

Barash, Cullen, Stoelting. *Clinical Anesthesia*, 2nd Edn. Chapter 30.

A 5. **A.** true **B.** false **C.** false **D.** false **E.** false

Cricoid pressure is Sellick's manoeuvre (Brian Sellick being a London anaesthetist). It involves 30–40 N of pressure on the cricoid cartilage which forms the only complete ring of the larynx and trachea. The cartilage is identified at C6 and the index finger is placed against it in the midline with the thumb and middle finger on either side. It is intended to protect against passive regurgitation and aspiration of stomach contents. It must be released during active vomiting to prevent oesophageal rupture.

Yentis, Hirsch, Smith. *Anaesthesia A to Z*. Butterworth Heinemann.

A. false **B.** false **C.** false **D.** false **E.** false

IVRA is a potentially lethal technique, and requires appropriate care and monitoring to be performed safely (see 'Paper Mask' starring Paul McGann). TWO IV cannulae are required, although neither need necessarily be 'large bore'. An IV cannula should be placed for resuscitation at a site remote from the limb to be blocked. A cannula will also need to be placed in the limb that is to be blocked. The limb should be adequately exsanguinated before a proximal cuff is inflated to twice the systolic blood pressure. In patients with uncontrolled hypertension, there is no guarantee that complete arterial occlusion will occur, and hence the technique is relatively contraindicated. However, allergic sensitivity to amide local anaesthetics and sickle cell disease are more absolute contraindications. Approximately 40–50 ml of local anaesthetic solution (prilocaine 1% or lignocaine <1%, NOT bupivacaine because of its cardiovascular toxicity) is injected into the limb slowly. Higher concentrations of LA may be inappropriate because of toxicity at these volumes (6 mg/kg maximum for prilocaine). A distal tourniquet may be inflated 10 min after the injection, and the proximal tourniquet deflated. This places the tourniquet over an anaesthetised area thus relieving tourniquet pain. Full monitoring should be employed. Irrespective of the length of the procedure, the tourniquet should not be deflated until >20 min have elapsed, to prevent washout of unbound local anaesthetic solution, preventing toxicity. Tourniquet pain frequently limits the duration of anaesthesia to less than 1 h.

Yentis, Hirsch, Smith. *Anaesthesia A to Z*. Butterworth Heinemann, 1993.

A. true **B.** false **C.** true **D.** false **E.** false

The mainstay of preoperative preparation is the institution of α-adrenergic blockade and the re-expansion of the circulating blood volume. This is usually undertaken over a 10 to 14-day period. Control of systemic blood pressure (to a maximum of 160/95 for 48 h before surgery), orthostatic hypotension (to a minimum of 80/50 on standing), nasal congestion and an increased frequency of bowel motions have all been advocated as signs of adequate α-adrenergic blockade prior to surgery. Increased body weight in combination with a reduction in the serum haematocrit (3–5%) usually indicates a satisfactory restoration of the circulating plasma volume. Although passive re-expansion is usually sufficient to achieve this, precipitous posture-related reductions in the systemic blood pressure may require the addition of intravenous fluid therapy.

Hutton, Cooper. *Guidelines in Clinical Anaesthesia*. Blackwell, Chapter 6.

A 8. A. false **B.** true **C.** true **D.** false **E.** false

Oral hypoglycaemic agents should be replaced by subcutaneous insulin and preferably prior to conception as they have been linked with an increased risk of teratogenicity. Tight glycaemic control is mandatory throughout pregnancy as foetal blood glucose is dependent on that of the mother and maternal insulin cannot cross the placenta. Insulin requirements may fall rapidly and unpredictably following delivery, so it is advisable to initiate an intravenous insulin infusion to cover the period of labour. Insulin requirements increase and the renal threshold for glucose falls with advancing pregnancy. Hence, blood rather than urine glucose should be tested regularly to guide insulin requirements. Epidural analgesia is particularly indicated for diabetic parturients. Not only does it limit the hyperglycaemic stress response to pain but also provides suitable anaesthesia for instrumental and operative delivery, which are more likely to occur in the diabetic mother. However, an adequate perfusion pressure across the placental bed must be maintained at all times as the foetus is particularly vulnerable to developing acidosis.

Murphy P. *Essays & MCQs in Anaesthesia and Intensive Care*, Chapter 9.

A 9. A. false **B.** false **C.** true **D.** true **E.** true

When a blood donation is made it must be stored correctly to both maximise its shelf-life and effectiveness when used. Blood is initially collected into bags containing an anticoagulant (CPD) solution and then cooled to a temperature of 4°C until used. Donated whole blood can be stored in this form for up to 3 weeks, but more commonly is centrifuged down to produce a red cell concentrate. (The platelet, plasma and white cell fractions are kept for further refinement and possible clinical use.) Plasma-reduced blood consists of red blood cells suspended

Answers

in a small volume of plasma (haematocrit 65–70%) which may, or may not, be depleted of leucocytes. It should be used within 24 h of preparation. Re-suspension of the red cell concentrate in a nutrient solution of saline, adenine, glucose and mannitol (SAG-M) will prolong its shelf life to 5 weeks. Red cells that have had all traces of leucocytes, platelets and plasma removed may be frozen with glycol to produce an almost indefinite storage time. These units are extremely expensive to prepare and are usually given only to those patients with rare blood groups or with antibodies against common blood group antigens. Cryoprecipitate is prepared from fresh frozen plasma. It contains higher concentrations than are found in plasma of fibrinogen, von Willibrand factor, factors VIII/XIII and fibronectin. It is valuable in the rapid reversal of the effect of fibrinolytic agents and in promoting haemostasis in various conditions where fibrinogen concentration is reduced. Dilutional thrombocytopaenia secondary to massive blood transfusion should be treated with platelet transfusion only if the platelet count is $<50 \times 10^9$/l and the patient is bleeding. The recovery of platelets 1 h after transfusion is 50–80% with a reduced half-life in the circulation of approximately 4 days. ABO blood group compatibility is not essential but preferable. In contrast, transfused fresh frozen plasma (FFP) must be ABO compatible. It contains normal plasma levels of clotting factors and its use should be confined to those patients with significant bleeding and laboratory evidence of coagulopathy.

Contreras M. *ABC of Transfusion*, 2nd Edn. BMJ Publishing.

A 10. **A.** false **B.** true **C.** true **D.** false **E.** true

The clinical features of foreign body aspiration are sudden onset of choking, dysphonia, coughing and stridor. There may also be decreased air entry and wheezing in the lung distal to the obstruction. On the chest radiograph the foreign body may be visible or there may be hyperinflation of the lung distal to the obstruction. The latter is often best seen on a film taken at the end of expiration. If the obstruction has been present for some time, partial or complete distal collapse of the lung may also be evident. The Stortz rigid bronchoscope has the advantage over the Negus bronchoscope of a side arm for attachment of the anaesthetic breathing system and superior optical characteristics.

Exam 1

Answers

The Negus, in contrast, has a tapered shape and a larger lumen that makes for the easier removal of an inhaled foreign body. Jet ventilation, utilising the Venturi principle, can be used with the Negus bronchoscope. Spontaneous ventilation is mandatory in respiratory obstruction, regardless of the underlying cause, unless the anaesthetist is certain that it will be possible to adequately ventilate the lungs of the paralysed patient. An inhalational induction with halothane (or sevoflurane) in oxygen is the induction technique of choice in infants and small children.

Hatch, Sumner, Hellman. *The Surgical Neonate: Anaesthesia & Intensive Care*, 3rd Edn. Edward Arnold, Chapter 4.

A 11. **A.** true **B.** true **C.** true **D.** true **E.** true

Extracorporeal shock wave lithotripsy is performed outside the operating suite. It involves both immersion and non-immersion techniques. Anaesthesia is required as electrohydraulic lithotripsy (water bath) is painful; the arrival of the focused shock wave at the skin/water interface releases energy which is dissipated at the skin. The shock waves are triggered from the ECG signal. If they are initiated during the RT interval, cardiac conduction disturbances occur manifesting as premature ventricular and atrial contractions as well as supraventricular tachycardia. This is resolved by initiating the shock 0.2–0.22 ms after the R wave during the absolute refractory period. Contrast material used in cerebral angiography can cross the blood-brain barrier and this may result in seizures. This may be due to direct toxicity or chemoreceptor trigger zone stimulation. Radiation therapy in children commonly involves anaesthesia as immobility is required. Radiation doses are in the range 180–250 rad per treatment, so personnel must leave the room. This means the patient and monitors can only be observed indirectly usually via closed circuit TV. MRI entails placing the patient in a magnetic field. Burns from the pulse oximeter have been described from heating of the probe in the MRI. CT scanner suites are often cooler than 25°C to allow for optimal functioning of the equipment. This may predispose to hypothermia under general anaesthesia especially in the paediatric population.

Barash, Cullen, Stoelting. *Clinical Anaesthesia*, 2nd Edn. Chapter 54.

12. **A.** true **B.** false **C.** true **D.** true **E.** false

Patients homozygous for sickle cell haemoglobin have HbSS and HbA, those heterozygous have HbAS in addition to HbA. Heterozygotes are normally asymptomatic unless exposed to extreme hypoxia.

Kumar, Clark. *Clinical Medicine*, 3rd Edn. Saunders, Chapter 6.

13. **A.** false **B.** true **C.** false **D.** true **E.** false

Topical anaesthesia using 4–10% cocaine applied to the nose should not exceed 3 mg/kg. As well as anaesthetising, it causes vasoconstriction. The epiglottis, base of tongue and mucosa down to the cords may be blocked by anaesthetising the superior laryngeal nerve. This can be performed by injection of local anaesthetic below the greater cornu of the hyoid bilaterally or by holding a local-anaesthetic-soaked pledget in the piriform fossa bilaterally, or simply by gargling anaesthetic solution. Trans-tracheal injection of anaesthetic blocks the trachea and larynx below the cords. It is best to ask the patient to breathe out fully before injecting as the resultant inspiration and coughing aids spread of anaesthetic. Nebulised 4% lignocaine has been used as the sole anaesthetic but it may not be as effective as a combination of techniques. Fibreoptic instruments are delicate. They consist of bundles of glass fibres each of which is encased in glass of different refractive index. The fibres are lubricated and flexible. Disinfectant passed into the scope may disrupt this lubrication. They should be cleaned soon after use to prevent crusting of secretions and according to the manufacturer's guidelines.

Yentis, Hirsch, Smith. *Anaesthesia A to Z*. Butterworth Heinemann.

14. **A.** false **B.** true **C.** false **D.** false **E.** false

Adverse drug reactions are classed as type A or B. Type A are dose-related extensions of pharmacological response and are common. Type B are not dose-related e.g. anaphylaxis. They are uncommon and do not yield responses which are an extension of the drugs actions. Initially anaphylaxis causes a drop in blood pressure or loss of pulse followed in a minority of cases by bronchospasm. Immediate treatment is discontinuation of the agent that triggered the response, airway maintenence with 100% oxygen and giving adrenaline and fluid. IV adrenaline should be titrated to response in doses of 50–100 μg aliquots, or with severe cardiovascular collapse up to 1 mg. The IM dose is 0.5–1 mg repeatable. Blood for tryptase should be taken approximately 1 h from the start of the reaction but not before the patient is safe. It is stored at −20°C in a plain bottle until sent to the lab. Later skin testing should be undertaken with all drugs used except volatiles. It is the responsibility of the anaesthetist to investigate and follow-up the patient.

Association of Anaesthetists of Great Britain & Ireland. *Suspected Anaphylactic Reactions Associated With Anaesthesia*, Revised Edn. 1995.

A 15. **A.** false   **B.** false   **C.** true   **D.** false   **E.** false

The coaxial Mapleson D is the Bain circuit. The fresh gas flow (FGF) runs through the narrow inner tube within the outer corrugated tubing. The integrity of the inner tube may be assessed as described by Pethick. If intact, with an inflated reservoir bag, when oxygen is flushed into the circuit a Venturi effect occurs at the patient's end leading to a decrease in the pressure in the circuit, and the bag deflates. A leak in the inner tube allows fresh gas to escape into the expiratory limb and the bag remains inflated. During controlled ventilation Bain and Sporel recommend the following FGF rates to maintain normocarbia with the Mapleson D: 2 L/min for infants less than 10 kg, 3.5 L/min for patients from 10–50 kg and 70 ml/kg for those over 60 kg. The Mapleson A is the Magill circuit. This is an efficient circuit during spontaneous ventilation. Rebreathing can be prevented if the FGF equals or exceeds the patient's minute ventilation. The Lack circuit is a coaxial version of the Magill, but remember that to prevent rebreathing the expiratory valve should not be screwed tightly open (it will then be able to stop flow from the expiratory limb during inspiration). During controlled ventilation the Mapleson A is inefficient and requires a FGF of 20 L/min to allow adequate CO_2 elimination in a 60-kg patient. The Mapleson F is the Jackson Rees modification of the Mapleson D. This is a T-piece with a reservoir bag and incorporates a relief mechanism for venting exhaled gases; this may be a valve or simply a hole in the bag. FGF may be humidified by allowing it to pass through an in-line heated humidifier.

Barash, Cullen, Stoelting. *Clinical Anesthesia*, 2nd Edn. Chapter 25.

A 16. **A.** true **B.** false **C.** true **D.** false **E.** false

The sixth cranial nerve may be compressed with increased intracranial pressure causing failure of lateral gaze, but a dilated pupil is due to compression of the third cranial nerve. Sensory fibres from the ophthalmic division of the fifth cranial nerve carry sensation from the tip of the nose. These pass through the superior orbital fissure. The pupil described is an Argyll Robertson pupil, which is small and irregular in size and accommodates but does not react to light.

A 17. **A.** false **B.** true **C.** true **D.** false **E.** false

Anticholinesterases are prosthetic (reversible, competitive short-acting inhibitors) or acid-transferring (forming a compound which may be irreversible or of intermediate duration). Effects are equivalent to cholinergic stimulation but the site and nature of the effect depends on the penetration of the drug administered. Drugs containing a quaternary ammonium group (neostigmine, pyridostigmine) are less likely to cause CNS effects because they are polar and cannot cross the blood-brain barrier and tend to be limited to muscarinic and peripheral nicotinic receptors. Lipid-soluble agents such as physostigmine and the organophosphates act on the central cholinergic receptors within the brain. In addition to NMJ effects, the anticholinesterases augment vagal effects, cause bronchial smooth muscle contraction and bronchial secretion, increase gut activity, cause pupillary constriction and improve aqueous outflow.

Anticholinesterases and anticholinergic drugs Nair VP, Hunter JM. *Continuing Education in Anaesthesia, Critical Care and Pain*. BJA Publications, October 2004, Volume 4, Number 5.

A 18. **A.** true **B.** true **C.** false **D.** true **E.** true

The regulation of aldosterone release is dependent on several factors other than angiotensin II, including potassium levels. The heart and vascular endothelium can activate angiotensinogen-using proteases other than ACE. Spironolactone can cause significant hyperkalaemia particularly when added to ACE inhibitors and digoxin. The addition of spironolactone to patients with severe heart failure (ejection fraction approximately 30%) taking ACE inhibitors and other diuretics improves mortality.

Inhibitors of the renin angiotensin system: implications for the anaesthesiologist. Licker M, Morel D. *Current Opinion in Anaesthesiology* 1998;11:323–326.
Weber K. Aldosterone and spironolactone in heart failure. *New England Journal of Medicine* 1999;341:10;753–755 and 709–717.

A **19.** **A.** false   **B.** true   **C.** false   **D.** false   **E.** false

Halothane has a blood gas solubility of 2.5 (enflurane is 1.9) and is 20% metabolised by the liver (enflurane is 2% metabolised and isoflurane is 0.2% metabolised). It has a MAC of 0.75, a molecular weight of 197.4 g, a boiling point of 50.2°C, an SVP of 241 mmHg and is non-flammable. It depresses respiration causing rapid shallow breathing and may cause postoperative sputum retention. It is a bronchodilator. It is negatively inotropic, but less so than enflurane. It also causes a bradycardia and is arrhythmogenic.

Barash, Cullen, Stoetling. *Handbook of Clinical Anesthesia*, 2nd Edn. Lippincott.

A **20.** **A.** false   **B.** true   **C.** false   **D.** false   **E.** true

Desflurane is an entirely fluorinated derivative of isoflurane which confers stability. It has a low potency with an MAC of 6%. Cyclopropane has an MAC value of 9.2%. Blood gas solubility of desflurane is 0.42. It has a boiling point of 23.5°C, but is heated to 39°C in the TEC 6 vapouriser. Its molecular weight is 168 g, which is lower than all the other currently available vapours (halothane = 197.4 g; enflurane and isoflurane = 184.5 g; sevoflurane = 200 g) and its vapour pressure at 20°C is 664 mmHg. It is stable with soda lime and biodegradability is minimal (approx 0.02%). Cardiovascular and respiratory effects are minimal. Uptake and elimination are similar to nitrous oxide.

Barash, Cullen, Stoetling. *Handbook of Clinical Anesthesia*, 2nd Edn. Lippincott.

A 21. A. false   **B.** false   **C.** false   **D.** false   **E.** true

Normal CSF pressure is 5–13 mmHg but the gradation on a manometer is in centimetres. Remember, mercury has a density 13.6 times that of water (giving the conversion factor for the height of the column). Tentorial herniation causes IIIrd nerve compression. Tonsillar herniation causes neck stiffness and Cheyne-Stoke breathing. Lundberg A (interval 5–20 min, ICP 50–100 mmHg) and B (interval about 1 min, ICP up to 50 mmHg) waves are always superimposed on an elevated ICP and indicate failed compensatory mechanisms. C waves (0.1 Hz up to 20 mmHg) may also be pathological but can occur in normal patients. Hypocapnia-induced cerebral vasoconstriction lessens demonstrably between 6 and 10 h but clinically often, more quickly. The frequency of severe raised intracranial pressure during Grade 3 and 4 encephalopathy, during fulminant hepatic failure and subsequent liver transplantation, makes ICP monitoring useful for cerebroprotection and prognosis.

Schubert A. *Clinical Neuroanaesthesia*. Butterworth Heinemann, 1996.

A 22. A. true   **B.** false   **C.** false   **D.** true   **E.** true

The renal system is apparently the only system where capillaries (glomerular) empty into arterioles (efferent) and then into peritubular and long vasa recta capillaries again. Angiotensin converting enzyme inhibitors cause a fall in GFR, in part, by causing relaxation of the efferent arteriole more than the afferent arteriole and so reducing glomerular pressure. NSAIDs do not influence glomerular filtration under normal circumstances but can cause significant loss of function if there is effective loss of circulating volume due to any cause. PGI2 and PGE2 are released during hypovolaemia and cause vasodilation that may protect the kidney from ischaemic damage. The symptoms of uraemia, anorexia, nausea, vomiting, lethargy, poor sleep and concentration and pruritis, occur late in loss of renal function, are caused by retained toxic products and are non-specific; Anaemia occurs earlier at around a GFR of 30 ml/min. The normal young adult renal blood flow is about 22% of cardiac output. RBF = Plasma flow/1 − haematocrit.

Ganong W. *Review of Medical Physiology*, 18th Edn. Appleton and Lange, 1997.
Gaskin G. *Medicine* 1999;275:1–4.
Harris K. *Br J Anaes* 1992;69:233–235.

A **23.** **A.** false **B.** true **C.** false **D.** true **E.** true

FEV_1 is reduced by an increased airway resistance. A low FEV_1/FVC ratio suggests an obstructive defect.

West. *Respiratory Physiology*, 4th Edn. Williams and Wilkins, Chapter 10.

A **24.** **A.** true **B.** true **C.** true **D.** false **E.** false

Respiratory quotient is the carbon dioxide output divided by the oxygen uptake in the basal state. The total amount of dissolved carbon dioxide in the body is approximately 120 L.

Stoelting. *Handbook of Pharmacology and Physiology in Anesthetic Practice*. Lippincott-Raven, Chapter 50.

A **25.** **A.** true **B.** true **C.** false **D.** true **E.** false

Peripheral neuropathic pain involves peripheral and central (spinal cord) sensitisation. A-β fibres carry sensations of touch and pressure and cannot activate dorsal horn pain paths. However, continuous A-β activity or dorsal horn disinhibition by other mechanisms may lower the threshold for appreciating a painful stimulus via these neurons. Schwann cells are not just axonal insulators. Injury causes these cells to secrete growth factors effecting changes in neuronal sodium channel and phenotypic expression. The AMPA (aminohydroxy-methylisoxazole-proprionic acid) receptor is the rapidly functioning receptor for glutamate, the main transmitter released in response to nociceptor activity. NMDA (N-methyl-*D*-aspartate) receptors, which are also activated by glutamate, require another stimulus to open. Phosphorylation removes a magnesium ion that blocks the channel under resting conditions. The subsequent decrease in threshold depolarisation in dorsal horn pain neurons is one cause of central sensitisation. Cholecystokinin (CCK) production increases from injured neurones and is an antagonist at opioid receptors. Sprouting of sympathetic nerve terminals around dorsal root ganglia is a possible mechanism for sympathetically maintained pain. A-β fibres may sprout into the dorsal horn after peripheral nerve injury producing an abnormal nociceptive input.

Woolf C, Mannion R. *Lancet* 1999:353;1959–1964.

A 26. **A.** false **B.** true **C.** true **D.** true **E.** true

It is essential to have a basic knowledge of pain pathways and common pain syndromes for the fellowship examination since this material is also often visited as a viva question. C fibres are involved in slow pain transmission, and unlike A delta fibres are unmyelinated. You should be able to score 5/5 on this question!

Stoelting. *Handbook of Pharmacology and Physiology in Anesthetic Practice.* Lippincott-Raven, Chapter 43.

A 27. **A.** true **B.** true **C.** false **D.** true **E.** false

A series in 1966 suggested survival after the onset of angina, syncope or heart failure was 5, 3 and 2 years respectively. Recent studies suggest that, if symptomatic, aortic stenosis is associated with an average survival of less than 2–3 years. Many clinicians will not proceed to valve replacement in asymptomatic patients despite investigation findings. Measurements may be misleading. Severe stenosis produces a trans-valvular pressure gradient of 50 mmHg in the presence of a normal cardiac output but a smaller gradient in a failing heart. A large patient with a valve area greater than 1.0 cm^2 may still have severe stenosis. Any drug that reduces coronary perfusion pressure during diastole can induce a vicious circle of ischaemia, failure and falling perfusion pressure usually managed urgently with vasoconstrictors. However, nitrates have been used in the medical management of angina associated with aortic stenosis and in the treatment of ischaemia under anaesthesia. Coronary dilatation, smaller left ventricular end diastolic size and increasing the diastolic aortic to left ventricular end diastolic pressure gradient may be responsible.

ACC/AHA Guidelines for the management of patients with valvular heart disease. *JACC* 32:5;1486–1588.

A 28. **A.** false **B.** true **C.** true **D.** true **E.** false

Squamous cell carcinoma is the commonest type of respiratory tract tumour. Adenocarcinomas are usually peripheral, often producing a sub-pleural mass.

Kumar, Clark. *Clinical Medicine*, 3rd Edn. Saunders, Chapter 12.

A 29. **A.** false **B.** true **C.** false **D.** false **E.** true

The normal portal venous pressure is 5–8 mmHg. β-blockers reduce portal venous pressure, are effective at reducing re-bleeding rates and can be used in primary prevention of bleeding in patients with known oesophageal varices. Obviously thay cannot be used in bleeding hypovolaemic patients. Terlipressin and vasopressin reduce splanchnic blood flow and portal pressure in bleeding varices but they both have significant coronary artery constrictor effects, which may be offset by simultaneous nitrate therapy. Octreotide has a better side effect profile and in some trials is as effective as emergency endoscopic control of bleeding but not superior. Therefore it is a useful adjunct and may prevent early re-bleeding while definitive endoscopic treatment is established. Constrictive pericarditis along with right heart failure, Budd-Chiari syndrome and veno-occlusive disease are rare, but important, causes of posthepatic portal hypertension.

Burroughs A. *Medicine* 27;1:70–74; Kumar P, Clark M. *Clinical Medicine*, 3rd Edn. Bailliere Tindall, 1994.

A 30. **A.** true **B.** true **C.** false **D.** true **E.** true

Cardiac troponin I and troponin T are components of the myocardial contractile apparatus. They are highly specific markers of myocardial necrosis and are normally undetectable. They are released in infarction and severe ischaemia as well as associated conditions which result in myocardial muscle damage e.g. myocarditis, pulmonary embolus, cardiac failure and renal failure. Serum levels take several hours to rise and peak at 12–24 h so admission values may be misleading. Values remain raised for up to 14 days so they are little use as monitors of acute re-infarction.

Cardiac troponins in chest pain. Hillis GS, Fox KA. *BMJ* 4th December 1999;319. http:\\www.bmj.com

A 31. **A.** false **B.** true **C.** true **D.** false **E.** false

Down's syndrome is often associated with endocardial cushion defects causing atrial and ventricular septal defects and abnormalities of the mitral and tricuspid valves. Coarctation of the aorta is usually at or just distal to the insertion of the ductus arteriosus.

Kumar, Clark. *Clinical Medicine*, 3rd Edn. Saunders, Chapter 11.

A **32.** **A.** true   **B.** true   **C.** false   **D.** true   **E.** true

Patients with Prader-Willi syndrome are hypotonic and usually obese.

Mather, Hughes. *A Handbook of Paediatric Anaesthesia*. Oxford University Press, Chapter 6.

A **33.** **A.** false   **B.** true   **C.** false   **D.** false   **E.** false

Hereditary angioneurotic oedema usually affects the face, upper airway, extremities and gut. Oedema is precipitated by tissue trauma, and dental extraction without prophylaxis is associated with life-threatening upper airway obstruction. Attacks are not reliably prevented or treated with adrenaline or steroids because they are predominantly mediated by complement, not histamine. Therefore, the recommended treatment for an attack is fresh frozen plasma or a C1-esterase concentrate. Regional anaesthesia has not proven dangerous. By contrast, some anaesthetists have counselled against tracheal intubation in case of trauma inducing oedema, although intubation has been accomplished safely.

Poppers P. *Canadian Journal of Anaesthesiology* 1987;34:76–78.

A **34.** **A.** true   **B.** false   **C.** false   **D.** false   **E.** true

Carotid endarterectomy is usually performed to reduce risk of stroke in patients with carotid stenosis. It can be performed using cervical plexus block, but is more commonly performed under general anaesthesia in the UK. Hypotension should be avoided at all times and direct intravascular monitoring of arterial blood pressure is mandatory. Hyperglycaemia has been implicated in contributing to cerebral ischaemic damage and thus glucose infusions should be avoided. Normocapnia is now advocated by most, although hypercapnia through hypoventilation had been advocated in the past to increase cerebral blood flow. This is now thought to increase the risk of cerebral steal. Carotid sinus stimulation during surgery can lead to hypotension and

Exam 1

Answers

bradycardia, and can be prevented by infiltration with local anaesthetic solution.

Yentis, Hirsch, Smith. *Anaesthesia A to Z*. Butterworth Heinemann, 1993.

A 35. **A.** true   **B.** true   **C.** true   **D.** true   **E.** true

Marfan's syndrome is caused by defects in the fibrillin protein. There is a broad phenotypic spectrum and many potential problems. Myopia, lens dislocation, retinal detachment and cataract are more common in Marfan's syndrome. Cystic lung disease makes spontaneous pneumothorax more common. Ventilation may be further impaired by kyphoscoliosis and pectus excavatum. Mitral valve prolapse and aortic root dilatation are the commonest cardiac lesions and ascending aortic dissection or heart failure due to chronic aortic regurgitation used to be the most frequent modes of death until prophylactic replacement was introduced. Patients with aortic root dilatation greater than 40 mm or family history of aortic dissection are at increased risk of dissection in pregnancy. A long narrow skull, high-arched palate and temporomandibular joint abnormalities may increase the difficulty of intubation.

Katz J *et al. Anaesthesia and Uncommon Diseases*, 3rd Edn. W.B. Saunders Philadelphia, 1990.
Gott V. *N Engl J Med* 1999;340:1307–1313.

A 36. **A.** true   **B.** true   **C.** true   **D.** true   **E.** false

Although acute shifts in potassium are more familiar, there are many causes of high potassium losses from the body such as a new ileostomy or chronic diarrhoea that deplete total intracellular stores. Pancreatic secretions are rich in bicarbonate. Fat malabsorption results in the formation of calcium 'soaps' in the gut and free oxalate that is usually complexed with calcium is reabsorbed predisposing to oxalate stones. Secondary hyperparathyroidism is secondary because of hypocalcaemia.

Zilva J, Pannell P, Mayne P. Clinical Chemistry in Diagnosis and Treatment, 5th Edn. Edward Arnold, 1988.

A. true **B.** false **C.** true **D.** true **E.** false

A right thoracotomy is performed during the Ivor Lewis procedure. 80% of colorectal cancers are found in the sigmoid and rectum.

Prys-Roberts, Brown. *International Practice of Anaesthesia*. Butterworth Heinemann, Chapter 115.

A 38. **A.** false **B.** true **C.** false **D.** false **E.** true

The Childs' classification is a method of risk assessment for cirrhotic patients undergoing major surgery. Pugh-Child's grading of the severity of liver disease incorporates clinical and biochemical measurements. 1, 2 or 3 points are scored for increasing abnormality in the following categories: Encephalopathy; Ascites; Serum bilirubin; Serum albumin and Prothrombin time. Cardiovascular effects of advanced liver disease are typically a high cardiac output and low systemic vascular resistance. In hepatorenal syndrome the kidneys cannot excrete sodium. Urine sodium concentration is less than 10 mmol/L.

Prys-Roberts, Brown. *International Practice of Anaesthesia*. Butterworth Heinemann, Chapter 73.

A 39. **A.** false **B.** true **C.** true **D.** true **E.** false

There is usually a single dominant anterior spinal artery supplemented by two smaller posterior arteries. There are anastomoses with branches from the aorta, intercostal and lumbar arteries with an important contribution made by a large vessel, the artery of Adamciewicz that arises variously in the thoracolumbar region. Hyperglycaemia results in worse neural damage in man and in experimental animal models. The early hazard of suxamethonium is well documented but the precise time at which it becomes contraindicated is contentious. Some authorities recommend 24 h. However, chronic denervation is also a well-documented cause of potentially dangerous potassium release associated with suxamethonium.

Webb A, Shapiro M, Singer M, Suter P. *Oxford Textbook of Critical Care*. Oxford University Press, 1999.

A 40.   **A.** false   **B.** false   **C.** true   **D.** true   **E.** true

Cement is a self-polymerising granular methyl methacrylate and a liquid monomer, used as a space-filling mortar. It transmits compressive loads from bone to prosthesis to bone. It is not glue. The odour of the liquid monomer, though pungent, is not a biohazard. The cement-bone interface is said to be better if there is no blood covering the cancellous bone as the cement is applied. For this reason, hypotensive anaesthesia has been shown radiographically to improve the quality of cement bone fixation by reducing bleeding from bone at the time cement is applied. However, hypotension and hypoxaemia may occur on insertion of the prosthesis due to the presence of the cement itself, rendering a hypotensive technique hazardous. The true cause of this is unknown. It may be directly cardiotoxic, allergic in nature or caused by vasodilation due to heating. Haemolysis releasing toxins, activation of the coagulation cascade or fat/air/debris emboli have also been proposed as theories. Risks are reduced by washing out the cavity with saline prior to cement insertion, venting the cavity, and filling it retrogradely to avoid air trapping.

Barash, Cullen, Stoelting. *Clinical Anesthesia*, 2nd Edn. Chapter 44.

A 41.   **A.** false   **B.** false   **C.** true   **D.** false   **E.** true

Fourier showed that any waveform may be represented by composites of sine-waves at harmonics of the fundamental frequency (in this case heart rate). If the amplitude and the shape of the arterial waveform are to be accurately recorded, 10 harmonics of the fundamental frequency (the heart rate) are required. The system must then be optimally damped, so that oscillations caused by the driving frequency being close to the resonant frequency of the recording system do not interfere too much with accuracy of both the waveform shape and the waveform amplitude. Critical damping is said to occur when the output waveform responds to change as rapidly as possible, without amplitude overshoot i.e. the system just fails to oscillate. Critical damping is represented by a damping coefficient of 1.0. Optimal damping occurs when the damping coefficient is 0.66. This represents the best compromise between accurate recording of the amplitude and accurate recording of the shape of the waveform. An overdamped waveform will record reduced systolic pressure and increased diastolic pressure, whilst the mean pressure will remain unaltered, and thus, the pulse pressure will be artefactually reduced.

Nimmo, Rowbotham, Smith. *Anaesthesia*, 2nd Edn. Blackwell Scientific Publications, Chapter 35.

A **42.** **A.** false **B.** true **C.** true **D.** true **E.** true

Trans-oesophageal echocardiography (TOE) is increasingly used as a perioperative monitor of myocardial function, cardiac output, ejection fraction, end-diastolic volume, air embolus and ischaemia. It is a very sensitive tool for detecting air embolus (although it may detect clinically insignificant quantities of air). Ischaemia is detected by the observance of regional wall motion abnormalities, although it is worth remembering that they may be caused by scarring, tethering of the myocardium or as normal variability.

Nimmo, Rowbotham, Smith. *Anaesthesia*, 2nd Edn. Blackwell Scientific Publications, Chapter 35.

A **43.** **A.** true **B.** false **C.** true **D.** false **E.** false

The prothrombin time tests the extrinsic and common coagulation pathways. It is performed using plasma, calcium, brain extract and phospholipid. The activated partial thromboplastin time (APTT) tests the intrinsic and common pathways. Plasma, phospholipid and calcium are added to kaolin. Normal value is 35–40 s. The activated clotting time (ACT) is a bedside test used commonly to measure the adequacy of heparin anticoagulation during cardiopulmonary bypass. It is performed by adding celite to whole blood, and timing fibrin formation. Normal values are 100–140 s, and values 3–4 times normal are considered adequate for cardiopulmonary bypass. The bleeding time is a bedside test of platelet function. A standard incision is made on the forearm, a sphygmomanometer cuff is inflated to 40 mmHg and the incision is dabbed every 30 s until the bleeding stops. Normal value is 2–9 min. The thromboelastograph (TEG) gives fairly rapid bedside information about speed of clot formation and strength of clot. It is commonly used in orthotopic liver transplantation.

Yentis, Hirsch, Smith. *Anaesthesia A to Z*. Butterworth Heinemann.

A 44. **A.** true **B.** false **C.** false **D.** true **E.** false

Normal spontaneous tidal volumes are possible whilst 80% of Ach receptors remain occupied by the neuromuscular blocker, it is therefore an insensitive indicator of reversal. Twitch height is difficult to measure objectively, hence the use of a train of four allowing comparative assessment of fade. Train of four becomes normal at 70–75% receptor occupancy. Sustained tetanus is possible at 70% receptor occupancy to a 50-Hz stimulus and 50% receptor occupancy for a 100-Hz stimulus – both are extremely painful! Hand grip, head lift and ETT-measured inspiratory pressure all appear normal at 50% receptor occupancy.

Miller. *Anesthesia*, 4th Edn.

A 45. **A.** true **B.** true **C.** false **D.** true **E.** true

Septal Q waves in I, aVL and V6 are normal. A Q wave in III is also a normal variant. Left atrial hypertrophy causes broad, bifid P waves. Peaked P waves are caused by right atrial hypertrophy.

Hampton. The *ECG Made Easy*, 4th Edn. Churchill Livingstone.

A 46. **A.** true **B.** true **C.** true **D.** true **E.** true

Infrared thermometers measure the amount of radiation emitted by a surface as a proportion of its known maximal emittance (emissivity). Temperature of the surface determines how close measured radiation of infrared comes to known emissivity. The Seebeck effect is a system used to measure temperature. At a junction of two dissimilar metals a small voltage is produced, the magnitude being proportional to the temperature at the junction. This type of junction is known as a thermocouple. A second junction completes the electrical circuit and generates another temperature-dependent voltage. To be used as a thermometer, one of the junctions is kept at a constant temperature and the other acts as the measuring probe. Small probes have smaller heat capacities.

Parbrook GD, Davis PD, Parbrook EO. *Basic Physics and Measurement in Anaesthesia*. Butterworth Heinnemann.

47. **A.** true   **B.** false   **C.** false   **D.** true   **E.** false

Fat Embolism Syndrome (FES) most frequently complicates long bone fractures but has also been described in a wide range of conditions, ranging from bone marrow transplantation to acute haemorrhagic pancreatitis and sickle cell crisis. A lot of patients remain asymptomatic despite a very high incidence of fat embolism following major trauma. In those who develop symptoms, isolated respiratory insufficiency in association with tachycardia and fever is probably the commonest manifestation. The chest X-ray may appear abnormal with bilateral, diffuse, non-specific shadowing of the lung fields but more frequently than not, arterial blood gas analysis reveals hypoxaemia in the absence of CXR changes. The classic triad of respiratory insufficiency, neurological dysfunction and petechial rash is only found in 1–5% of patients with FES. The rash is pathognomonic of FES and typically affects the conjunctivae, oral mucosa and skin covering the axilla and neck. It is thought to be due to capillary occlusion by fat globules or thrombocytopaenia. Thrombocytopaenia, raised fibrinogen degradation product (FDP) levels, hypocalcaemia and a fall in haematocrit may all occur but are non-specific findings. In severe cases of FES, ischaemic changes and a right ventricular strain pattern may appear on the ECG. Widespread mechanical occlusion by fat globules of the pulmonary microvasculature is responsible for the initial rise in pulmonary vascular resistance. Localised tissue damage then follows, resulting in platelet accumulation and activation with the release of powerful vasoactive mediators. Fat globules may then gain access to the systemic arterial circulation via 'shunts' recruited in the face of an increasing pulmonary vascular resistance.

Murphy P. *Essays & MCQs in Anaesthesia and Intensive Care*. Edward Arnold, Chapter 19.

48. **A.** true   **B.** true   **C.** false   **D.** true   **E.** true

An intra-aortic balloon pump may be required in order to maintain myocardial diastolic perfusion, whilst surgery might be necessary for acute valvular dysfunction. α-Adrenoceptor agonists will only serve to worsen cardiogenic shock and should not be used. Nitroprusside can be used to rapidly vasodilate and thereby offload the patient, whilst amiodarone may be needed for any arrhythmias.

Oh T. *Intensive Care Manual*, 4th Edn. Butterworth Heinemann, Chapter 15.

A **49. A.** false **B.** true **C.** true **D.** false **E.** false

All acute coronary syndromes should receive immediate treatment with 'MONA' therapy (**M**orphine or diamorphine titrated IV, **O**xygen at high flow, **N**itroglycerine sublingually, **A**spirin 300 mg orally). Dihydropyridine calcium channel blockers such as nifedipine are not recommended because the resultant vasodilatation and hypotension may precipitate reduced coronary artery perfusion and a reflex tachycardia that increases myocardial oxygen demand, and therefore ischaemia. Indications for thrombolytic therapy include presentation within 12 h with chest pain suggestive of an MI and ST segment elevation >0.2 mV in 2 adjacent chest leads or >0.1 mV in 2 or more limb leads, dominant R waves and ST depression in V1–3 (posterior MI), or new-onset LBBB. Presentation 12–24 h after onset with continuing pain +/− ECG evidence of an evolving infarct is also an indication. Absolute contraindications to thrombolysis include: previous haemorrhagic stroke, CVA within 6 months, active internal bleeding (menses excluded) and aortic dissection. Streptokinase is given as 1.5 million units in 100 ml saline over 1 h. Alteplase is given as 15 mg IV bolus followed by 0.75 mg/kg over 1 h then 48 h of heparin therapy. Reteplase is given as 10 units IV bolus followed by 10 units IV bolus after 30 min then 48 h of heparin therapy.

Resuscitation Council (UK). *Advanced Life Support Provider Manual*, ISBN 1–903812–05–4.

A **50. A.** false **B.** false **C.** false **D.** false **E.** true

Clostridium tetani is a gram positive, non-invasive organism which does not confer natural immunity, and so, following an infection, the patient will still have to undergo a vaccination programme. Although tetanolysin is produced, it appears to have no clinical effects. The clinical symptoms and signs are caused by a toxin called tetanospasmin, which affects the inhibitory neurones via the glycinergic terminals in the spinal cord and the GABA terminals in the brain.

Oh T. *Intensive Care Manual*, 4th Edn. Butterworth Heinemann, Chapter 47.

A 51. **A.** false **B.** true **C.** true **D.** true **E.** true

Severe sepsis is a multi-system disorder. Do not be seduced by terms you have never heard of. As far as we know perivascular thromboembolism does not exist as a medical term!

Oh T. *Intensive Care Manual*, 4th Edn. Butterworth Heinemann, Chapter 61.

A 52. **A.** true **B.** false **C.** true **D.** false **E.** true

Hypothermia is defined as a core temperature of below 35°C. The 'J' wave is a relatively constant finding below 33°C but is at the junction of the QRS complex and the T wave. Atrial fibrillation is a common arrhythmia in hypothermia. Ventricular fibrillation is common below 28°C and asystole below 20°C. Respiratory drive does not cease until around 24°C. Initially renal blood flow increases which leads to a diuresis and haemoconcentration. Rewarming may unmask this relative hypovolaemia.

Craft TM, Nolan JP, Parr MJA. *Key Topics in Critical Care*, 1st Edn. BIOS Scientific Publishers.

A 53. **A.** false **B.** false **C.** true **D.** true **E.** false

Botulism is a rare but potentially fatal disease. It is caused by a Gram positive bacillus. Most infections are caused by food-borne organisms. A preformed exotoxin is absorbed from the gut and carried to nerve endings where it binds irreversibly. In severe cases a progressive flaccid paralysis occurs. Tendon reflexes are normal or decreased.

Oh T. *Intensive Care Manual,* 4th Edn. Butterworth Heinemann, 1997.

A 54. **A.** false **B.** true **C.** false **D.** true **E.** false

Ventilation strategies can be controversial. Intrinsic PEEP is measured at the end of expiration. An increase in airway obstruction, ventilatory rate or tidal volume can increase pulmonary hyperventilation. Hypotension during mechanical ventilation is usually due to dynamic hyperinflation (intrinsic or auto-PEEP), sedation or pneumothorax. These are often aggravated by hypovolaemia and so will be helped by fluids, but treatment should be aimed at the cause. Myopathy can be a severe problem in ventilated asthmatics. Aetiology is not clear and although neuromuscular blocking drugs have been implicated the problem can occur without their use.

Oh T. *Intensive Care Manual*, 4th Edn. Butterworth Heinemann, 1997.

A 55. **A.** true   **B.** true   **C.** true   **D.** true   **E.** true

Although not used commonly, most ventilation modes can be used non-invasively. There is increasing interest in non-invasive ventilation on intensive care and respiratory units.

Oh T. *Intensive Care Manual*, 4th Edn. Butterworth Heinemann, 1997, Chapter 27.

A 56. **A.** true   **B.** false   **C.** true   **D.** true   **E.** false

CO poisoning may result from inhalation of car exhaust fumes, smoke from fires or fumes from faulty heating equipment. The amount of carboxyhaemoglobin (COHb) formed depends on the inspiratory concentration and the duration of exposure. CO has an affinity for haemoglobin of 240–250 times that of O_2 and once bound it dissociates very slowly. Dissociation is enhanced by increasing the partial pressure of O_2, firstly by inspired fraction and in severe cases by increasing ambient pressure as well using a hyperbaric chamber. Normal COHb levels in the blood are 0.3–2%, rising to 6% in cigarette smokers. At levels above 60% CO poisoning can present with coma. Neurological and psychiatric symptoms occur more frequently after CO poisoning than in the general population. Standard pulse oximetry is ineffective as a means of assessment of degree of poisoning since 'cherry red' COHb is misread as oxyhaemoglobin. Bench oximetry employs an additional light source which enables this extra species of haemoglobin to be differentiated from the normal variants. PaO_2 is unaffected by CO poisoning but at normal ambient pressure the contribution of plasma-dissolved O_2 to overall O_2 delivery is less than 5%, so it is misleading as a prognostic indicator.

Yentis, Hirsch, Smith. *Anaesthesia A to Z*. Butterworth Heinemann, 1993.

57. **A.** false **B.** true **C.** true **D.** false **E.** true

Streptococcal pneumonia is the commonest cause of pneumonia in the previously fit. *H. influenza* is only common in those with pre-existing lung disease. Cold agglutinins occur in approximately 50% of patients with mycoplasma pneumonia.

Kumar, Clark. *Clinical Medicine*, 3rd Edn. Saunders Chapter 12.

58. **A.** true **B.** false **C.** true **D.** true **E.** true

Metabolic acidosis is caused either by an increased production of metabolic acids such as in tissue hypoxia or diabetic ketoacidosis, an inability to utilise oxygen (histotoxic hypoxia) such as in cyanide poisoning, following the ingestion of acids (salicylate poisoning), following the loss of bicarbonate-rich fluid from the gastrointestinal tract (e.g. diarrhoea), following the inability to excrete hydrogen ions (renal failure) or following the administration of drugs (e.g. acetazolamide). Guillain-Barre syndrome is a postinfection polyneuropathy which progresses to produce respiratory impairment and a respiratory acidosis.

Yentis, Hirsch, Smith. *Anaesthesia A to Z*. Butterworth Heinemann.

59. **A.** true **B.** false **C.** false **D.** false **E.** true

In addition to pregnancy and liver failure, a low plasma urea:creatinine ratio is also typically seen in over-hydration and in patients receiving a low protein diet. This contrasts with the following clinical situations where, providing there are no complicating factors, the plasma urea tends to be elevated out of proportion to the plasma creatinine: cardiac failure, diuretic therapy, gastrointestinal haemorrhage and high protein intake with or without an associated increase in protein catabolism (corticosteroid therapy, trauma, infection etc.). Plasma urea and creatinine rise in parallel in chronic and established acute renal failure.

Murphy P. *Essays & MCQs in Anaesthesia and Intensive Care*. Edward Arnold, Chapter 17.

A 60. **A.** true   **B.** true   **C.** true   **D.** false   **E.** false

Perioperative nutritional support should be started early both in patients with pre-existing malnutrition and in those patients who are likely to have a prolonged postoperative recovery complicated by inadequate oral intake. Enteral feeding is less expensive than parenteral feeding, more complete and associated with a lower incidence of complications and morbidity. Small intestinal motility and function are maintained in the postoperative period; therefore, feeding tubes that bypass the stomach allow enteral feeding to be initiated in the immediate postoperative period. Total parenteral nutrition is indicated for high protein and energy requirements, malabsorption and intractable diarrhoea. Energy is provided in the form of carbohydrate and fat. Carbohydrate calories are more efficient than lipid calories but in high concentration (>10%) are irritants to veins. Fat solutions, by contrast, are non-irritant and so offer an alternative energy source in a smaller volume. The usual daily protein requirement is 1–2 g/kg. This is administered as a mixture of essential and non-essential amino acids of which 25% should consist of essential amino acids. Specific dietary substrates have been used for their specific effects on metabolic and immune function. Glutamine is an amino acid that facilitates nitrogen transport and is the major fuel for enterocytes. Arginine improves macrophage and natural killer cell cytotoxicity, stimulates T-cell function and modulates nitrogen balance.

Goldhill, Strunin. *The High-risk Surgical Patient*. Bailliere Tindall, Chapter 13. Craft TM, Nolan JP, Parr MJA. *Key Topics in Critical Care*. BIOS Scientific Publishers.

A 1. **A.** true **B.** true **C.** false **D.** true **E.** false

Inhalational agents including nitrous oxide are cerebral vasodilators and increase cerebral blood flow and intracranial pressure (ICP). Mannitol is an osmotic diuretic, which in the dose of 0.5 g/kg, increases serum osmolality and causes a diuresis. This decreases ICP within 5 min of starting the infusion. However there is a transient hypervolaemia that may increase surgical bleeding. Steroids in head injury do not influence ICP or overall outcome. Anticonvulsants, usually phenytoin, are required with depressed skull fractures with dural penetration and following acute subdural haematoma. If fitting persists diazepam or phenobarbitone may be used. They also help reduce the metabolic rate of the brain, which occurs during convulsions. When trying to reduce raised ICP, normal fluid balance and electrolytes should be the aim. Dehydration does not assist.

Aitkenhead, Smith. *Textbook of Anaesthesia*, 2nd Edn. Churchill Livingstone, Chapter 38.

A 2. **A.** true **B.** true **C.** false **D.** false **E.** false

Looped cables made of conducting material can lead to current induction, but the use of fibreoptic systems overcomes this. Non-invasive blood pressure monitoring is straightforward as long as the monitor is kept out of the magnetic field (or a non-ferromagnetic system is used) and it has nylon connections.

Prys-Roberts, Brown. *International Practice of Anaesthesia*. Butterworth Heinemann, Chapter 117.

A 3. **A.** false **B.** false **C.** true **D.** false **E.** false

Read the question carefully – you are asked how many mmols are present in 500 ml, not per litre. 'Hartmann's solution for injection' is more correctly referred to as 'compound sodium lactate intravenous infusion'. Virtually every anaesthetic room stocks it, so you need to know that it contains sodium chloride 0.6%, sodium lactate 0.25%, potassium chloride 0.04% and calcium chloride 0.027%. This equates to Na^+ 131 mmol/L, Cl^- 111 mmol/L, lactate 29 mmol/L, K^+ 5 mmol/L, Ca^{2+} 2 mmol/L.

British National Formulary

A 4. **A.** false **B.** true **C.** true **D.** true **E.** false

Inhaled foreign bodies usually lodge in the right main bronchus because of its more vertical angle and greater width. CXR may reveal unilateral overinflation if the object is acting as a 'ball valve', preventing lung deflation, although distal atelectasis is more commonly seen. Removal requires rigid bronchoscopy for adequately sized forceps to be used. N_2O should be avoided to prevent overexpansion if distal air trapping has occurred. Positive pressure ventilation may force the object into more distal airways.

Yentis, Hirsch, Smith. *Anaesthesia A to Z*. Butterworth Heinemann, 1993.

A 5. **A.** true **B.** true **C.** false **D.** false **E.** false

Laparoscopic cholecystectomy requires the introduction of gas (CO_2) into the peritoneal cavity. This carries the risk of puncture of any hollow viscus/organ, and the stomach should be aspirated via an orogastric tube to remove any build-up of anaesthetic gases that may have occurred during positive pressure ventilation using a facemask prior to the commencement of surgery. As pressure rises in the peritoneum venous return is initially improved slightly, then reduced due to caval compression (>4 kPa) leading to hypotension secondary to reduced cardiac output. Measured blood pressure depends upon the site of measurement and is a function of cardiac output and vascular resistance. Therefore higher intra-abdominal pressures can cause direct abdominal aortic compression and upper body hypertension. Laparoscopic diathermy would need to be avoided if N_2O was used as the insufflating gas, as there is a risk of explosion. CO_2 is universally used to avoid this risk. Gas flow rates should not exceed 4 L/min, and total gas volume should not exceed 5 L.

Yentis, Hirsch, Smith. *Anaesthesia A to Z*. Butterworth Heinemann, 1993.

A. true **B.** true **C.** false **D.** true **E.** false

Down's syndrome (trisomy 21) results from the presence of an extra chromosome 21. Associated congenital abnormalities include congenital heart disease (ASD, VSD, Tetralogy of Fallot), duodenal atresia, airway difficulties leading to an increased incidence of difficult intubation and mental retardation. Atlantoaxial instability occurs more commonly in patients with Down's syndrome. Hypotonia is commonly present.

Yentis, Hirsch, Smith. *Anaesthesia A to Z*. Butterworth Heinemann, 1993.

A 7. **A.** false **B.** false **C.** true **D.** false **E.** true

Essential or idiopathic hypertension accounts for approximately 90% of all cases of hypertension in the Western world. Patients are frequently asymptomatic and have cardiac outputs similar to age-matched normotensives. Their increased blood pressure is therefore caused by differences in vascular resistance and compliance. Hypertension is a major risk factor for coronary artery disease, stroke and cardiac failure. With adequate preoperative treatment, perioperative mortality and incidence of stroke is greatly decreased but there is a much less dramatic effect on the incidence of myocardial infarction. The hypertension optimal treatment (HOT) study indicates that the treatment goal is to reduce pressure to 140/85 mmHg in the long term. The BNF recommends the following approach to hypertension in general : immediate therapy for patients with BP >220/>120 mmHg; confirmation over 1–2 weeks then treat for patients with BP 200–219/110–119 mmHg; confirmation over 3–4 weeks then treatment for patients with BP 160–199/100–109 mmHg. Considerable evidence now exists that with diastolic blood pressures of up to 110 mmHg, painstaking perioperative monitoring and pharmacological control of the blood pressure are probably more important than preoperative antihypertensive therapy in terms of decreasing the incidence of subsequent cardiovascular complications. (An exception to this is in patients undergoing carotid endarterectomy, where inadequately controlled hypertension preoperatively is associated with postoperative neurological deficits.) Patients with diastolic blood pressures >120 mmHg have been found to exhibit exaggerated haemodynamic responses to anaesthesia and to be at a

Exam 2

Answers

significantly increased perioperative risk of subendocardial ischaemia and stroke. The upstroke of the arterial waveform reflects the contractility of the myocardium, while the downstroke provides information on the compliance and resistance of the systemic vascular bed.

Hypertension: pathophysiology and treatment. Foex P, Sear JW. *Continuing Education in Anaesthesia, Critical Care & Pain.* BJA publications, Volume 4, Number 3, June 2004.
Murphy P. *Essays & MCQs in Anaesthesia and Intensive Care.* Edward Arnold, Chapter 1.
Hutton, Cooper. *Guidelines in Clinical Anaesthesia.* Blackwell, Chapter 1.

A 8.   **A.** true   **B.** true   **C.** true   **D.** true   **E.** false

Amniotic fluid embolism is a rare (1 in 80,000 pregnancies) but often fatal condition (mortality rate approximately 80%) and is the commonest cause of sudden maternal death during the course of labour or delivery. Typically the patient is older, multiparous and has a tumultuous labour. For amniotic fluid to enter the circulation there must be a tear in the membranes. This may range from artificial rupture of the membranes to rupture of the uterus. Consequently, both amniotic fluid and air embolism can occur at LSCS, especially if the placenta is incised. Delayed respiratory depression is an ever-present risk when epidural opioids are used but is less likely to occur when lipophilic agents such as fentanyl and diamorphine are used. The risk of pulmonary aspiration of gastric contents under regional anaesthesia is greatly reduced but can still occur in the presence of a very high neuroaxial block. Intragastric acidity should therefore be controlled with antacid therapy regardless of whether LSCS is performed under general or regional anaesthesia. With modern anaesthetic techniques, the induction of anaesthesia to delivery interval has no bearing on foetal outcome. In contrast, the uterine incision-to-delivery (U-D) interval is an important factor and if prolonged by more than 3 min under spinal anaesthesia has been shown to result in a higher incidence of low umbilical artery pH values and lower 1 min Apgar scores in the newborn.

Moir, Thorburn. *Obstetric Anaesthesia & Analgesia*, 3rd Edn. Bailliere Tindall, Chapter 9.
Murphy P. *Essays & MCQs in Anaesthesia and Intensive Care.* Edward Arnold, Chapter 10.

A. true **B.** true **C.** false **D.** false **E.** true

Haemophilia 'A', an X-linked recessive deficit of factor VIII, affects males almost exclusively. Plasma levels of factor VIII will vary between individuals resulting in differing severities of the disease. If the plasma level is greater than 10% of normal, then abnormal bleeding is unlikely to occur – unless surgery is performed. Factor VIII concentrate is therefore given to maintain levels around 15% for normal, healthy day-to-day living. Prior to surgery, this dose will need to be increased to ensure a plasma factor VIII activity of at least 30% or preferably higher. Factor VIII deficiency predominantly affects the intrinsic clotting system. This is reflected in a prolongation of the partial thromboplastin time while the prothrombin time remains normal. Platelet numbers/function and fibrinogen concentration, all are normal. Tranexamic acid and aminocaproic acid, both inhibitors of fibrinolysis, have been used to reduce bleeding in haemophiliacs undergoing dental extractions. In addition, DDAVP (a vasopressin analogue) given in advance of a surgical procedure has been shown to increase plasma levels of factor VIII and may reduce the subsequent requirement for factor VIII concentrate and cryoprecipitate.

Contreras M. *ABC of Transfusion*, 2nd Edn. BMJ Publishing.

A 10. **A.** true **B.** true **C.** false **D.** true **E.** true

The normal maintenance fluid volume requirement (hourly) for a fit child can be calculated using the formula: (4 ml/kg up to 10 kg) + (2 ml/kg for the second 10 kg) + (1 ml/kg for each kg thereafter). In the short term, fluid composition is based upon a need for 2 – 3 mmol/kg per day of both sodium and potassium. There are potential problems with glucose homeostasis in infants and small children due to a combination of reduced liver glycogen stores and impaired gluconeogenesis. In health, a standard solution of 4% glucose/0.18% saline with an addition of 10 mmol potassium chloride to every 500 ml bag is usually satisfactory to meet both the metabolic and electrolyte requirements of the smallest infants. It must be remembered, however, that neonates and sick children are vulnerable to hypoglycaemia and that electrolytes may therefore need to be infused in 10% or even 15% glucose solutions. The regular use of Dextrostix (or BM stix) is an important safeguard of

Exam 2

Answers

normoglycaemia. Urine production of 0.3 – 0.5 ml/kg/h in a fit neonate and >0.5 ml/kg/h in older children suggests adequate hydration. The normal circulating blood volume in infants and children is estimated as 80 ml/kg. There is a greater degree of cardiovascular reserve in response to haemorrhagic shock in children and a loss of up to 15% of the circulating blood volume is usually well tolerated without the need for blood transfusion.

Hatch, Sumner, Hellmann. *The Surgical Neonate: Anaesthesia and Intensive Care*, 3rd Edn. Edward Arnold, Chapter 2.

A 11. **A.** true **B.** false **C.** false **D.** true **E.** true

The electrically induced grand mal seizure produced by ECT is responsible for the therapeutic effect rather than the electrical stimulus. The seizure may last several minutes and consists of a short 10- to 15-s tonic phase followed by a more prolonged clonic phase. The seizure causes a wide range of physiological effects. These include initial bradycardia and hypotension with later tachycardia, arrhythmias, hypertension and increased systemic and myocardial oxygen consumption. There is increased cerebral blood flow, elevated intracranial pressure and elevated intraocular and intragastric pressure.

Barash, Cullen, Stoelting. *Clinical Anaesthesia*, 2nd Edn. Chapter 54.

A 12. **A.** false **B.** true **C.** true **D.** false **E.** false

MAC or minimum alveolar concentration is an unfortunate term. It is conceptually easier to understand if it is regarded as minimum alveolar PARTIAL PRESSURE (MAPP). After all, a conventional vaporiser merely divides down SVP (saturated vapour pressure) to a workable anaesthetic partial pressure using a variable bypass or splitting ratio. MAC and MAPP conveniently coincide when concentrations are compared with partial pressures (kPa) at sea level where ambient pressure is approximately 100 kPa. Variations in inspired concentration or ambient pressure both give rise to changes in alveolar partial pressure of the inhaled agent, but the standard 'MAPP' quoted at sea level will remain valid within the range of ambient pressures used clinically (up to 6 atmospheres). However, even if the required inspired partial pressure remains constant at altitude, the apparent MAC

(N.B. CONCENTRATION) of an agent will appear to have risen because the fall in overall ambient pressure will have necessitated an increase in the fractional concentration of the agent to maintain the required partial pressure (Dalton's law of partial pressures). James and White tested Fluotec Mark II and Dräger Vapor halothane vaporisers at sea level, at 5,000-ft and 10,000-ft altitude. At any given setting the delivered percentage of halothane increased with altitude; however, its partial pressure remained constant. Therefore, when these devices are used at a given vaporiser setting, anaesthetic will be delivered at a constant potency regardless of altitude. The TEC 6 vaporiser is specifically designed to deliver desflurane. To overcome the difficulty of unpredictable vaporisation at 20 °C (desflurane has a boiling point of 23.5 °C), the vaporiser is electrically heated to maintain a constant 39 °C in the vaporisation sump. Here, ambient pressure is maintained at 2 atmospheres. Downstream, pressure is autoregulated to maintain a pressure of 1.1 atmospheres at a fresh gas flow of 10 L/min. Therefore, unlike contemporary variable-bypass vaporisers, the Tec 6 vaporiser requires manual adjustments of the concentration control dial at altitudes other than sea level to maintain a constant partial pressure of anaesthetic. Since it is working at its own pressure, altitude does not affect its output, and it will accurately deliver the dialled volumes percent of desflurane but this does not equal an accurate partial pressure of anaesthetic. To compensate for the reduction in partial pressure, the set concentration on the dial must be increased to maintain the required anaesthetic partial pressure. For example, at an altitude of 2,000 m, the anaesthetist would have to manually increase the concentration control dial from 10 to 12.8% to maintain the required anaesthetic partial pressure.

Miller. *Anesthesia*, 4th Edn. Chapters 9 and 71.

A 13. **A.** false **B.** false **C.** true **D.** false **E.** false

Phaeochromocytomas may secrete adrenaline and/or noradrenaline and may even secrete dopamine. Patients usually present with headache, psychosis, palpitations and hypertension. Cardiomyopathy and glucose intolerance occur. Preoperative preparation includes initial oral α-antagonists e.g. phenoxybenzamine, doxazosin, then β-blockade if the patient remains tachycardic. Initiation with the latter may exacerbate hypertension because of antagonism of β_2-mediated vasodilation in muscle. Perioperatively, catecholamines can be released by tumour handling. Sodium nitroprusside, phentolamine, GTN, prazosin and magnesium sulphate have all been used to control hypertension. β-blockers or antiarrhythmics can control tachycardia. Following removal, fluid and phenylephrine or dopamine can be used to maintain pressure.

Yentis, Hirsch, Smith. *Anaesthesia A to Z*. Butterworth Heinemann.

A **14.** **A.** true **B.** true **C.** false **D.** true **E.** false

In volume depleted patients in the left lateral position epidural anaesthetic leads to improved placental perfusion by up to 75%. The total body clearance of amides is prolonged and repeated administration can cause higher blood levels than in non pre-eclamptics. There is an increased sensitivity to vasopressors necessitating reduced dosage. General anaesthetics in pre eclamptics can be hazardous. Intubation can be difficult due to swollen tongue, epiglottis or pharynx. Magnesium sulphate prolongs the duration of non-depolarising muscle relaxants through its action on the myoneural junction. The use of a peripheral nerve stimulator is recommended.

Barash, Cullen, Stoelting. *Clinical Anesthesia*, 2nd Edn. Chapter 46.

A **15.** **A.** false **B.** false **C.** false **D.** true **E.** false

The Carlens tube is passed into the left main bronchus. It has a carinal hook aiding placement but which may hinder passage through the glottis. The Robertshaw tube has wider lumina side by side. Left and right versions are available as well as small, medium and large sizes. The Bryce–Smith tube is similar to the Carlens but has no hook. It also has a larger bronchial portion. The Brompton Pallister tube is passed into the left main bronchus. It has one tracheal cuff and two bronchial cuffs in case of damage to one. One has no pilot. Left-sided tubes are usually preferred because of the risk of inadequate ventilation of the right upper lobe with use of right-sided tubes. Exceptions are for sleeve resection of the left bronchus, left pneumonectomy for lung transplantation or to isolate infection.

Yentis, Hirsch, Smith. *Anaesthesia A to Z*. Butterworth Heinemann.

A. true   **B.** false   **C.** false   **D.** true   **E.** false

The aortic and pulmonary valves are semilunar valves and prevent backflow of blood into the ventricles during diastole. All the heart valves open and close passively and possess three cusps except the mitral valve, which has only two cusps. The semilunar valves are heavier, thicker and unlike the mitral and tricuspid valves are not supported by chordae tendineae connected to papillary muscles. Their greater mass means that they open and shut more sluggishly than the AV valves. Closure of the AV valves gives rise to the first heart sound. Closure of the pulmonary and aortic valves causes the (sometimes split) second heart sound. A pathological third heart sound may be heard in mid diastole and is said to be caused by blood flowing with a rumbling motion into the almost-filled ventricle.

Guyton AC. *Textbook of Medical Physiology*. Saunders, Chapter 13.

A 17. **A.** true   **B.** true   **C.** false   **D.** false   **E.** true

Thiazides act on the distal convoluted tubule to inhibit sodium and chloride reabsorption. The initial antihypertensive effect is thought to be due to decreased plasma volume although in the long term there may be a reduction in SVR. The primary mechanism of β-blockers is thought to be inhibition of β-mediated renin release and subsequent reduction in angiotensin 1 and 2 levels. Baroreceptor sensitivity is also increased. Noradrenaline release within the sympathetics is reduced by blockade of presynaptic β_2-receptors. Then there are the conventionally recognised myocardial effects on contractility and rate. Selective α-agonists such as prazosin and doxazosin act at the α-1 receptor to reduce catecholamine-mediated vasoconstriction. Phenoxybenzamine and phentolamine bind to both α_1- and α_2-receptors causing a reflex tachycardia by inhibiting reuptake of noradrenaline (α_2 mediated). Calcium channel blockers do act at L-type calcium channels leading to vasodilatation and negative inotropy. The dihydropyridines (nifedipine, amlodipine) act peripherally, whereas the non-dihydopyridines (verapamil, diltiazem) have actions in the conducting system and can produce bradycardias with β-blockers. The ACE inhibitors competitively inhibit conversion of

Exam 2

Answers

angiotensin 1 to angiotensin 2 in the lung and this reduces aldosterone release.

Kimpson P, Howell S. The physiology of the control of blood pressure and antihypertensive drugs. *Bulletin 25* (May 2004). The Royal College of Anaesthetists.

A **18.** **A.** false **B.** true **C.** false **D.** true **E.** true

11 5-HT receptor subtypes have been identified. All types of 5-HT receptors are located in the gastrointestinal tract. 5-HT$_1$ and 5-HT$_2$ receptors are believed to mediate enhanced gastrointestinal motility associated with carcinoid syndrome. However, the 5-HT$_2$ antagonists have no effect on bowel motility in normal healthy volunteers. 5-HT$_3$ receptors are located on enteric and splanchnic nerves mediating neuronal depolarisation. Administration of 5-HT to these receptors results in enhanced gastrointestinal tract motility. Ondansetron and granisetron fail to prevent this effect but gastroprokinetic properties are not common to all drugs of this type. 5-HT$_3$ antagonists have been found to reduce the rewarding effects associated with the abuse of heroin, cocaine, nicotine and amphetamines.

Hindle AT, Recent developments in the physiology and pharmacology of 5-HT. *BJA* September 1994;73:3.

A **19.** **A.** false **B.** true **C.** false **D.** true **E.** false

Enflurane is relatively non-irritant to the respiratory system. It has a blood gas solubility of 1.9, a MAC of 1.65, a boiling point of 56.5°C, a molecular weight of 184.5 g (= isoflurane, its isomer) and an SVP of 175 mmHg. It causes rapid shallow breathing without much increase in secretions. It causes hypotension mainly by decreasing cardiac contractility but it also decreases peripheral vascular resistance and causes a reflex tachycardia.

Barash, Cullen, Stoetling. *Handbook of Clinical Anesthesia*, 2nd Edn. Lippincott.

A **20.** **A.** true **B.** true **C.** false **D.** false **E.** false

Desflurane is more stable than isoflurane. Its blood-gas partition coefficient is lower than isoflurane at 0.42 (versus 1.4) which means more rapid alterations in depth of anaesthesia and more rapid recovery. Its effects on the cardiovascular systems are probably equivalent to isoflurane. Metabolism is 0.02% (compared with 0.2% for isoflurane) and it is not defluorinated to any extent. Both vapours are too pungent to make them suitable for gaseous induction.

Barash, Cullen, Stoetling. *Handbook of Clinical Anesthesia*, 2nd Edn. Lippincott.

A 21. **A.** true **B.** true **C.** true **D.** true **E.** true

ATP, adenosine, CGRP and acetylcholine are all released from vesicles from the neurone and have receptors on the muscle side of the neuromuscular junction (NMJ). Multiple effects have been observed and purposes proposed. A nerve fibre and its fascicule of muscle fibre is a motor unit. Physiologically during fasciculation the motor unit fibres contract synchronously but different motor units are contracting abnormally. Fibrillation occurs when muscle fibres contract asynchronously and is indicative of an NMJ of muscle fibre origin. The foetal γ subunit of the nicotinic NMJ receptor switches to adult ϵ subunit production when the nerve fibre makes contact with the muscle. Chronic denervation results in the production of foetal receptors again which are expressed all over the muscle and can cause large releases of potassium in response to suxamethonium stimulation. Vagal postsynaptic muscarinic receptor block by pancuronium is not the only mechanism of tachycardia but includes presynaptic activity at muscarinic receptors on sympathetic nerves that facilitates noradrenaline release.

Bowman W in *Recent Advances in Anaesthesia and Analgesia,* Adams A, Cashman J (eds). Churchill Livingstone, 1998.

A 22. **A.** true **B.** true **C.** false **D.** false **E.** false

The foetus exists in a comparatively hypoxic environment compared to the neonate. Blood is oxygenated in the placenta and passes through the single umbilical vein to the foetal IVC. Blood going to the head is about 67% saturated compared to blood beyond the mixing point of the ductus arteriosus which is 60% saturated. The left shift of the foetal oxyhaemoglobin dissociation

Exam 2

Answers

curve and the higher haemoglobin concentration aid oxygen transfer and transport. There is a considerable placental shunt so umbilical venous blood does not attain full saturation and this is mixed with equal volumes of the foetal systemic venous return in the inferior vena cava. Indomethacin is typically used to aid closure of a PDA. Prostaglandins maintain patency. Non-steroidal anti-inflammatory drugs should not be given in the third trimester of pregnancy. The change from foetal to neonatal circulation requires a drop in pulmonary vascular resistance associated with lung inflation. The neonate normally does this by generating negative inspiratory pressures of between $-40\,cmH_2O$ and $-100\,cmH_2O$. To inflate and 'recruit' lung volume during resuscitation it is recommended to use 5 or 6 'inflation' breaths that are sustained for 2 s at 30–40 cmH$_2$O before ventilating at 30–40 breaths/min if needed. The foetus is prone to 'ion trapping' by virtue of its lower blood pH which aids the diffusion of the lipid-soluble unionised fraction of local anaesthetic drugs across the placenta.

Ganong W. *Medical Physiology.* Appleton and Lange, 1995.
Wood M, Wood A. *Drugs in Anesthesia*, 2nd Edn. Williams and Wilkins, 1990.
Advanced Paediatric Life Support, 2nd Edn. BMJ Publishing Group, 1997.

A 23. **A.** false **B.** true **C.** false **D.** true **E.** true

Parasympathetic effects are effected via the cranial and sacral outflow tracts and the vagus. All autonomic preganglionic neurons are cholinergic. Parasympathetic postganglionic neurons are also cholinergic. Effects of stimulation include: miosis (contraction of the iris); ciliary muscle contraction (for near vision); decrease in heart rate, contractility and conduction velocity; arteriolar dilatation; bronchiolar contraction; bronchial gland stimulation; GI sphincter relaxation and increased motility and secretion; gall bladder contraction; pancreatic endocrine and exocrine secretion; urinary sphincter relaxation and detrusor contraction and erection.

Ganong WF. *Review of Medical Physiology*, 10th Edn. Lange, Chapter 13.

A 24. **A.** true **B.** false **C.** false **D.** true **E.** false

Most of the decrease in blood pressure between the arteries and veins occurs in the arterioles. Pulsus paradoxus is an exaggerated decrease in the systolic blood pressure during inspiration.

Traube–Hering waves are cyclical increases and decreases in blood pressure that may reflect changes in the reflex activity of baroreceptors.

Stoelting. *Handbook of Physiology and Pharmacology in Anesthetic Practice.* Lippincott-Raven, Chapter 44.

A 25. A. false   **B.** true   **C.** true   **D.** false   **E.** true

Bradykinin is produced locally at the site of trauma. Substance P is an excitatory transmitter.

Stoelting. *Handbook of Physiology and Pharmacology in Anesthetic Practice.* Lippincott-Raven, Chapter 43.

A 26. A. true   **B.** false   **C.** false   **D.** true   **E.** true

It has been suggested that a significant contributory component to neural irritation in back pain is chemical. Inflamed discs or the release of the contents of the nucleus pulposus result in the release or activation of phospholipases particularly A2. This can produce prostanoid inflammatory mediators by the release of arachidonic acid. Therefore it is possible to have root irritation without compression. Nerves that are touched by prolapsed discs do not always produce pain and vertebral abnormalities alone are not a perfect guide to the cause of clinical symptoms. The involvement of the S1 root by an L5/S1 disc classically produces pain in the lateral side of the leg, foot, and lateral toes.

Rawal N. *Management of Acute and Chronic pain.* BMJ Books, 1998.

A 27. A. true   **B.** false   **C.** true   **D.** false   **E.** false

The main causes of CRF are glomerulonephritis, diabetes mellitus, hypertension, cystic disease and pyelonephritis. FBC commonly reveals a normochromic normocytic anaemia of about 8 g/dl due to uraemia affecting erythropoiesis. INR and APTT are usually normal. Platelet function is impaired by uraemia leading to prolonged bleeding time. DDAVP 0.3 μg/kg is infused to improve platelet function if bleeding is a problem. Residual renal function is best protected by avoiding hypotension and hypovolaemia/dehydration and drugs such as NSAIDs and enflurane. Sevoflurane is okay within normal MAC limits. Many patients benefit from perioperative saline infusion to reduce perioperative falls in renal artery perfusion. Potassium-containing solutions are generally avoided because of the increased incidence of hyperkalaemia. Hyperkalaemia is further exacerbated by use of suxamethonium and acidosis. Gastric emptying is delayed and increased gastric acidity multiplies the risk of aspiration pneumonitis. Other considerations: AV shunts should be protected from trauma (including NIBP cuffs), wound healing is impaired, timing of haemodialysis and calcium levels may be lower than normal.

Allman, Wilson. *Oxford Handbook of Anaesthesia*. OUP 2001, Chapter 5.

A **28.** **A.** true   **B.** false   **C.** true   **D.** true   **E.** false

Pulmonary hypertension has been defined as a mean PAP >15 mmHg or systolic PAP >30 mmHg at rest. The early rise in $PaCO_2$ is a consequence of worse ventilation-perfusion matching after the release of hypoxic pulmonary vasoconstriction by O_2 therapy and inadequate ventilatory compensation by the patient. The onset of pulmonary hypertension in middle life in scoliotic patients is often associated with nocturnal hypoventilation. Type III phosphodiesterase inhibitors may be useful especially if maintaining right ventricular preload with fluid is also exacerbating tricuspid regurgitation. These drugs improve right ventricular contractility, lusitropy and reduce pulmonary vascular resistance. Type V phosphodiesterase inhibitors such as sildenafil are used as systemic vasodilators.

Yentis, Hirsch, Smith. *Anaesthesia A–Z*. Butterworth Heinemann, 1995.
Sykes K in *Cardiovascular Physiology* Priebe H–J, Skarvan K (eds). BMJ Publishing Group, 1995.
Keogh B in *Clinical Anesthesia* Goldstone J, Pollard B, (eds). Churchill Livingstone, 1996.

A **29.** **A.** true   **B.** false   **C.** true   **D.** true   **E.** false

Child's classification of liver failure was initially used to determine outcome for patients undergoing portosystemic shunting procedures but has been extended to other hepatobiliary procedures. Spontaneous bacterial peritonitis occurs in approximately 10% of patients with ascites. Chronic liver disease is associated with pulmonary and systemic shunting. It is possible to distinguish acute tubular necrosis from hepatorenal syndrome with urine and blood analysis but pulmonary artery catheterisation has been advocated to distinguish hypovolaemia.

Kumar P, Clark M (eds). *Clinical Medicine*, 3rd Edn, Bailliere Tindall, 1994; White H, Caldwell C in *Intensive Care Medicine*, 4th Edn. Irwin R, Frank C, Rippe J (eds), 1999.

A 30. A. false **B.** true **C.** true **D.** false **E.** true

Viral p24 core antigen may be detected for 8–10 weeks following infection. The CD4 molecule is the cellular receptor for HIV. Seroconversion following a needlestick with HIV-infected blood occurs in approximately 0.3% of cases.

Kumar, Clark. *Clinical Medicine*, 3rd Edn. Saunders, Chapter 1

A 31. A. true **B.** true **C.** false **D.** true **E.** false

Multiple sclerosis is acquired most commonly between 15 and 40 years of age and genetic factors are involved in the aetiology. Suxamethonium may cause hyperkalaemia, and muscle atrophy may reduce the requirement for non-depolarising agents. Urinary incontinence and sexual impotence may occur early while tremor and spasticity are later findings. Stress and temperature may exacerbate the condition. Platelet aggregation may be increased. There is an increased incidence of epilepsy.

Nimmo, Rowbotham, Smith. *Anaesthesia*, 2nd Edn, Volume 2.

A 32. A. false **B.** true **C.** false **D.** false **E.** true

Motor neurone disease (MND) causes degeneration of motor neurones in the spinal cord, cranial nerves, motor nuclei and cortex. It does not affect the cerebellum or sensory system. Immunoglobulin is of no benefit.

Kumar, Clark. *Clinical Medicine*, 3rd Edn. Saunders, Chapter 18.

A 33. A. true **B.** true **C.** true **D.** false **E.** true

Hypothyroidism and its sequelae are often clinically subtle but important in the perioperative period. Hypothyroidism becomes more likely with increasing age after radioactive iodine. It is not unusual to find 'a block and replace regimen' for the management of hyperthyroidism. After the first year 3% of patients who have received radioactive iodine therapy for hyperthyroidism will become hypothyroid per year. Hypothyroidism and associated hypercholesterolaemia are a part of the pathogenesis of ischaemic heart disease. Patients with ischaemic heart disease require very careful gradual introduction of thyroxine in case of precipitating angina or myocardial infarction. Severe illness results in the inhibition of peripheral type I 5'deiodinase with a resulting fall in T3 and rise in inactive reverse-T3. This is part of the 'sick euthyroid syndrome.'

Franklyn J, Weetman A. *Medicine* 1998;25(4):20–28.

A 34. A. false **B.** true **C.** false **D.** false **E.** false

Berry aneurysms are commonest at the junction of the anterior cerebral and anterior communicating arteries. Vasospasm occurs in 70% of patients with a peak incidence at 7 days and surgery has the worst outcome during this time. The benefit of early intervention (0–3 days) is that around 30% of patients will not survive to late surgery (11–14 days). Unruptured aneurysms <10 mm in diameter have a risk of rupture of less than 0.05% per year. The current mortality and morbidity related to surgery greatly exceeds the 7.5-year risk of rupture. Prophylactic surgery is not currently recommended. Deliberate systolic hypertension between 150 and 240 mmHg has been used to treat postoperative vasospasm as part of 'hypertensive, hypervolaemic, haemodilution' therapy.

Mayberg M *et al. Circulation* 1994;90:2592–2605.
The International Study of Unruptured Intracranial Aneurysms Investigators. *N Engl J Med* 1998;339:1725–1733.

A 35. A. true **B.** true **C.** true **D.** true **E.** false

This was the rate in the North American Symptomatic Carotid Endarterectomy Trial (*N Engl J Med* 1998;339:1415–1425) and the European Carotid Surgery Trial (Lancet 1998;351:1379–1387). A Javid shunt still represents a severe stenosis and increases the risk of embolic events. Bilateral damage to chemoreceptors is almost inevitable because carotid atheroma is focused on the bifurcation near the carotid bodies. The treatment of asymptomatic stenosis is controversial. Three trials have failed to show any benefit. The Asymptomatic Carotid Atherosclerosis Trial did not show a reduction in disabling stroke or death. After CABG major neurological disability occurs in approximately 6% of patients with asymptomatic carotid stenosis, a rate similar to the perioperative risk of carotid endarterectomy. In general patients with asymptomatic carotid disease are considered at low risk for stroke and may undergo CABG without prior carotid endarterectomy.

Schubert A. *Clinical Neuroanaesthesia*. Butterworth Heinemann, 1997.
Stoneham M, Knighton J. *Br J Anaesth* 1999;82:910–919.

A 36. **A.** true   **B.** false   **C.** false   **D.** true   **E.** true

A Blalock-Taussig shunt is an anastomosis between subclavian artery and pulmonary artery, performed for conditions in which there is decreased pulmonary blood flow (e.g. pulmonary stenosis). The Rashkind procedure is the creation of an atrial septal defect by pulling the inflated balloon of a cardiac catheter through the foramen ovale.

Mather, Hughes. *A Handbook of Paediatric Anaesthesia*. Oxford University Press, Chapter 7.

A 37. **A.** true   **B.** true   **C.** true   **D.** false   **E.** true

Widening of the QRS complex occurs when the serum sodium falls to approximately 115 mmol/L. If bladder perforation occurs, it is likely to be extraperitoneal.

Prys-Roberts, Brown. *International Practice of Anaesthesia*. Butterworth Heinemann, Chapter 116.

A 38. **A.** true   **B.** false   **C.** false   **D.** true   **E.** true

Carcinoma of the stomach is relatively common but the colon and rectum are the commonest sites of GI cancer. It is particularly common in Japan and typically affects the 50- to 70-year age group. Incidence is higher in patients with type A blood and in patients with pernicious anaemia. 1% arises from chronic gastric ulcers. AFP is a marker for some ovarian, testicular and hepatic carcinomas. 90% of gastric cancers are adenocarcinomas.

McLatchie. *Oxford Handbook of Clinical Surgery*. Oxford Medical Publications, Chapter 16. Ellis, Calne. *Lecture Notes in General Surgery*. Blackwell, Chapter 22.

A 39. **A.** true **B.** false **C.** true **D.** false **E.** true

The thyroid isthmus may need to be retracted or divided during a surgical tracheostomy. It is recommended that tracheostomies be made through the second and third tracheal rings because higher approaches increase the likelihood of subglottic stenosis. Identifiable stenosis may occur after approximately one third of surgical tracheostomies but the majority do not cause clinical problems. Tracheostomies may be created by incision only, the removal of a disc of cartilage or the elevation of a flap of cartilage (although this technique is thought associated with a higher rate of stenosis). The removal of a disc or flap may make early reinsertion more reliable, but loss of the skin and strap muscle track with oedema and bleeding may still occur. An early change of tracheostomy is not usually required but one author has recommended that changes should not be attempted before 72 h. The fact that prolonged endotracheal intubation influences tracheostomy complications may confound statistics related to tracheostomy in ITU patients.

Surgery of the upper airway. Banerjee *et al*. *Baillieres Clinical Anaesthesiology 9*, Number 2, pp 317–335. Bailliere Tindall, 1999. Percutaneous dilatational tracheostomy: method, indications, contraindications and results. Walz M. *Current Opinion in Anaesthesiology* 1997;10:101–105. Cuschieri A, Gilies G, Moossa A. *Essential Surgical Practice*, 2nd Edn. Wright Publications, 1998.

A 40. **A.** true **B.** true **C.** false **D.** false **E.** false

The Mallampati classification originally only had 3 groups. The positive predictive value is the percentage of patients predicted to be difficult who are difficult. Unfortunately the sensitivity of the Mallampati test is approximately 50% and the number of false negative difficult intubations matches the number correctly identified. A grade C protrusion predicts almost certain difficult laryngoscopy.

Calder I in *Anaesthesia and Intensive Care for the Neurosurgical Patient*
Walters F *et al.* (eds). Blackwell Scientific Publications 1994.
Goldstone J *et al.* Handbook of Clinical Anaesthesia. Churchill Livingstone,
1996.

A **41.** **A.** false **B.** true **C.** false **D.** true **E.** true

When measuring the pulmonary capillary wedge pressure, the
catheter tip should be in West's zone III of the lung, to avoid
measuring distal airway pressure. High applied positive end-
expiratory pressure can exceed left atrial pressure, thus
erroneously raising the measured PCWP. There should be no
major disturbance to the pulmonary venous vasculature between
the tip of the catheter and the left atrium; hence, a left atrial
myxoma would alter the PCWP (although a right atrial myxoma
would not!) There should be no significant gradient between the
left atrium and the left ventricle if the PCWP is to represent the
LVEDP. Mitral stenosis would cause such a gradient, whereas
pulmonary stenosis would not.

Nimmo, Rowbotham, Smith. *Anaesthesia*, 2nd Edn. Blackwell Scientific
Publications, Chapter 35.

A **42.** **A.** false **B.** true **C.** true **D.** false **E.** false

Clinical monitoring of the degree of recovery of neuromuscular
function after the administration of neuromuscular-blocking
drugs is notoriously unreliable. Tests such as force of hand-
squeeze, tongue protrusion and ability to maintain a sustained
(>5 s) head lift from the pillow are all used. Of these, the head
lift is the most reliable. The use of nerve stimulators provides
more accurate assessment of the recovery of neuromuscular
function. The respiratory muscles are less sensitive to
neuromuscular blockers than the small muscles of the hand,
hence if the ulnar nerve is used to monitor blockade, and
recovery at this site is complete, respiratory insufficiency is very
unlikely. Equally, diaphragmatic movement can still occur when a
nerve stimulator demonstrates complete paralysis of a peripheral
muscle. Double burst stimulation requires two 60 ms bursts of
tetanic stimulation 0.75 s apart. Double burst stimulation is more
sensitive at detecting fade than the train of four ratio. Currents
of up to 60 mA are required for skin electrode stimulation of

peripheral nerves. Current should be limited to 80 mA because of the risk of electrical hazard.

Nimmo, Rowbotham, Smith. *Anaesthesia*, 2nd Edn. Blackwell Scientific Publications, Chapter 35.

A 43. A. true   **B.** true   **C.** false   **D.** true   **E.** false

Mixed venous oxygen saturation (SvO_2) must be measured from the right ventricle or the pulmonary artery, as superior and inferior vena caval saturations are different, and mixing occurs in the heart. SvO_2 is related to arterial O_2 content, cardiac output and oxygen consumption (which depends on the oxygen extraction ratio of different tissues). Normal is 75%. In acute haemorrhage, the arterial O_2 content falls, so the SvO_2 falls. In blood transfusion the arterial oxygen content rises, so SvO_2 rises. When peripheral shunting occurs (i.e. sepsis), the O_2 extraction ratio of peripheral tissue falls, so the SvO_2 rises.

Yentis, Hirsch, Smith. *Anaesthesia A to Z*. Butterworth Heinemann.

A 44. A. true   **B.** false   **C.** false   **D.** false   **E.** true

The compact Wright respirometer is useful for measuring tidal volumes. Volume measurement is achieved by monitoring the continuous rotation of a vane. It is inaccurate for continuous flow measurement and tends to over-read at high volumes because of inertia. Moisture can cause the gears to stick, which is less of a problem with the electronic version.

Parbrook GD, Davis PD, Parbrook EO. *Basic Physics and Measurement in Anaesthesia*. Butterworth Heinnemann.

A 45. A. false   **B.** true   **C.** false   **D.** false   **E.** true

The 'critical temperature' is the temperature above which a substance cannot be liquefied, however much pressure is applied. The 'pseudo-critical temperature' is the temperature below which a gas mixture may separate into its constituents. The critical temperature of nitrous oxide is 36.5°C. The filling ratio is the mass of gas in a cylinder divided by the mass of water that the empty cylinder could hold. The term 'vapour' is used to describe a substance that has left the liquid phase below its critical temperature (i.e. could still be liquefied by pressure) while a 'gas' is above that temperature and can no longer be liquefied by pressure alone.

Parbrook GD, Davis PD, Parbrook EO. *Basic Physics and Measurement in Anaesthesia*. Butterworth Heinnemann.

A 46. **A.** true **B.** false **C.** false **D.** true **E.** true

Absolute humidity is the mass of water vapour present in a given volume of gas. Relative humidity is the ratio of mass of water to the mass required to saturate the volume of gas at that temperature. The hair hygrometer measures relative humidity with accuracy between 30 and 90%. The hair gets longer as humidity rises, and the hair length controls a pointer moving over a scale. The wet and dry bulb thermometer measures the effect of latent heat of vaporisation (which can only occur at relative humidity less than 100%). Regnault's hygrometer consists of a silver tube containing ether. Air is blown through the ether and the resultant cooling leads to condensation on the tube. The temperature at which condensation occurs is called the 'dew point'. This represents the temperature at which the ambient air is fully saturated. For the same mass of water vapour relative humidity decreases with temperature. At 20°C the SVP of water is 2.4 kPa. At 37°C the SVP of water is 6.3 kPa.

Parbrook GD, Davis PD, Parbrook EO. *Basic Physics and Measurement in Anaesthesia*. Butterworth Heinnemann.

A 47. **A.** false **B.** false **C.** false **D.** true **E.** true

Lignocaine raises the threshold and energy requirements for defibrillation and is associated with postdefibrillation asystole. There is some evidence that the potent α-adrenergic stimulants are as effective as adrenaline (epinephrine). Although not widely advocated, vasopressin 40 μg is considered by some an effective alternative to adrenaline 1 mg and has the advantage of longer duration of action (20 min). Sodium bicarbonate should not be used routinely but only in prolonged arrests as it causes sodium overloading and hyperosmolality, paradoxical cerebral acidosis, myocardial depression and metabolic alkalosis with tissue deprivation of oxygen. It should only be used if ventilation of the lungs can be increased to clear the resultant increased production of carbon dioxide. Bretylium initially causes the release of norepinephrine (which results in a transient increase in blood pressure, heart rate and ventricular excitability) followed by vasodilatation. The antiarrhythmic effects of bretylium are similarly biphasic with an initial decrease of the duration of the action potential and effective refractory period followed by an increase. It should be noted that the use of bretylium is not currently recommended within ALS algorithms (2004).

Sasada M, Smith S. *Drugs in Anaesthesia and Intensive Care*, 2nd Edn. Oxford Medical Publications.
Oh T. *Intensive Care Manual*, 4th Edn. Butterworth Heinemann, Chapter 7.
Resuscitation Council (UK), *ALS Guidelines*. January 2004.

A 48. A. false **B.** false **C.** false **D.** true **E.** true

In early shock autoregulation ensures that GFR is well preserved but oliguria occurs due to antidiuretic hormone (ADH) and aldosterone secretion. Despite a reduction in pulmonary blood flow, PaO_2 is often initially well maintained by an increase in respiratory rate and minute volume. Catecholamines, glucagon and glucocorticoid secretion all contribute to insulin resistance. Neurogenic shock most commonly results from trauma to the cervical spine.

Oh T. *Intensive Care Manual*, 4th Edn. Butterworth Heinemann, Chapters 14 and 15.

A 49. A. false **B.** false **C.** false **D.** false **E.** false

In ARDS lung injury is inhomogeneous and compliance in various parts of the lung varies from near normal to markedly reduced. Mortality is somewhere between 50–60% and the majority of patients die from multiple organ failure with ARDS, rather than from their hypoxaemia. Those patients who do survive usually only have mildly impaired pulmonary function. Although used as one of the accepted treatment strategies, reverse ratio ventilation has not been shown to improve outcome and its use remains debatable.

Oh T. *Intensive Care Manual*, 4th Edn. Butterworth Heinemann, Chapter 29.

A 50. A. true **B.** true **C.** true **D.** true **E.** false

Clonidine, magnesium, metronidazole and benzylpenicillin have all been used successfully as part of the management of tetanus. Hyperbaric oxygen is probably of little value.

Oh T. *Intensive Care Manual*, 4th Edn. Butterworth Heinemann. Chapter 47.

A 51. A. true **B.** false **C.** false **D.** false **E.** true

LPS is an endotoxin, part of the outer membrane of Gram-negative bacteria, which can act as an initiator of septic shock. Nitric oxide has a pivotal role in the development of septic shock and in causing the vasodilatation, but along with PAF, is not a cytokine.

Oh T. *Intensive Care Manual*, 4th Edn. Butterworth Heinemann. Chapters 61 and 85.

A 52. A. false **B.** false **C.** true **D.** true **E.** true

The sepsis-related terms have been carefully and precisely defined by consensus. Systemic inflammatory response syndrome (SIRS) occurs following a wide range of clinical insults but requires the presence of 2 or more of the following conditions: temperature $>38°C$ or $<36°C$, heart rate >90 beats/min, respiratory rate >20 breaths/min or $PaCO_2 <4.3\,kPa$, white blood count $>12,000$ or $<4,000$ cells/mm^3 or $>10\%$ immature forms. Sepsis is the systemic response to infection as defined by the presence of 2 or more of the SIRS criteria. Severe sepsis is sepsis associated with hypoperfusion, hypotension or organ dysfunction. Septic shock is sepsis-induced hypotension, (systolic blood pressure $<90\,mmHg$, or a reduction of $>40\,mmHg$ from the baseline, or the need for vasopressors) despite adequate fluid resuscitation, along with the presence of perfusion abnormalities. Interleukin-1 and interleukin-8 are proinflammatory cytokines triggered by an initial insult such as infection. Interleukin-6 and interleukin-10 are anti-inflammatory mediators that exert negative feedback on the inflammatory process.

Craft TM, Nolan JP, Parr MJA. *Key Topics in Critical Care*, 1st Edn. BIOS Scientific Publishers.

A **53.** **A.** true **B.** true **C.** false **D.** false **E.** true

In diabetic ketoacidosis a large sodium deficit (e.g.
300–450 mmol) and potassium deficit (3–5 mmol/kg) occurs.
Anion gap is increased, 13–17 mmol/L is within the normal range.
Glycosuria causes an osmotic diuresis but ketonuria contributes
up to 50% of the osmotic diuretic load.

Oh T. *Intensive Care Manual*, 4th Edn. Butterworth Heinemann, 1997.

A **54.** **A.** true **B.** true **C.** true **D.** true **E.** false

Fat embolism is most often seen in orthopaedic trauma but there
are many other associations. Parenteral feeding rather than
enteral feeding is an association.

Oh T. *Intensive Care Manual*, 4th Edn. Butterworth Heinemann, 1997, Chapter 31.

A **55.** **A.** false **B.** true **C.** true **D.** false **E.** false

APACHE I has 34 physiological variables. This was reduced to 12
in APACHE II. APACHE III includes a modified GCS. This
assessment tool is used to compare systems and cannot be used
to accurately predict individual patient outcome.

A **56.** **A.** true **B.** true **C.** false **D.** false **E.** true

Factors associated with an increased mortality in patients with
community-acquired pneumonia include: age over 60 years,
respiratory rate >30 breaths/min, diastolic blood pressure
<60 mmHg, new atrial fibrillation, lung contusion, underlying
chronic disease, urea >7 mmol/L, white cell count <4 or >20,
albumin <35 g/L, PaO_2 <60 mmHg, multiple lobes involved on
the chest X-ray and staphylococcal infection.

Oh T. *Intensive Care Manual*, 4th Edn. Butterworth Heinemann, 1997,
Chapter 33.

A **57.** **A.** false **B.** true **C.** false **D.** true **E.** false

Although *Escherichia coli* is a normal gut commensal, *E. coli* 0157
is a toxic variant that was first reported as a human pathogen in
1982. Case reports have steadily risen in number from 50 in 1985

to 1,050 in 1995. *E. coli* 0157 multiplies naturally in the intestines of cattle, and has recently been found in sheep. It does not cause animal symptoms. Calves are particularly likely to be *E. coli* 0157 carriers. Human infection is most likely to occur via contamination of ground beef and unpasteurised milk. Paddling pools and lakes have been documented as a source of infection (probably via human or animal diarrhoea in unchlorinated water). Haemolytic uraemic syndrome is the commonest cause of ARF in children in the Western world. The syndrome comprises of haemolytic anaemia, low platelet count and renal failure. The commonest form occurs in children and is preceded by a diarrhoeal illness. The majority of cases are associated with verocytotoxin producing *E. coli*. Prognosis is good, mortality being around 3–7%. 15–40% have long-term renal impairment. Other complications include thrombotic thrombocytopaenic purpura with CNS involvement, mainly in adults and associated with a poor prognosis. The Scottish outbreak in 1996 involved 479 reported cases and caused 20 deaths.

H.U.S.H. (Haemolytic Uraemic Syndrome Help). UK *E. coli* support group.

A 58. **A.** false   **B.** false   **C.** false   **D.** true   **E.** true

Drowning is the third most common cause of accidental death in children in the UK. When the victim is first submerged, apnoea occurs and the heart rate slows because of the diving reflex. As apnoea continues, hypoxia causes tachycardia, a rise in the blood pressure and acidosis. Anywhere between 20 s and 3 min later a break point is reached and breathing occurs. Fluid is then inhaled but on touching the glottis causes immediate laryngospasm and a secondary apnoea. The latter eventually gives way to involuntary respiratory movements, which in turn leads rapidly on to cardiac arrest and death. Death frequently results from asphyxia secondary to severe laryngospasm without large volumes of liquid being aspirated into the lungs. Children who survive because of interruption of this chain of events not only require therapy for near drowning, but also assessment and therapy for hypothermia, injury and electrolyte imbalance. However, the latter is rarely seriously altered regardless of whether the child has been submerged in salt water or fresh water. In contrast to fresh water, salt water tends to remain in the alveoli and exert an osmotic effect, drawing fluid into the lungs from the intravascular compartment. Attempts at aspirating inhaled liquid from the lungs to limit this effect are usually unsuccessful. Most children who do not recover have been submerged for more than 3–8 min. However, if the time to the first gasp occurs between 1 and 3 min after the start of basic life support and/or the rectal temperature recorded on arrival at hospital is less than 33°C, the chances of survival are increased. (The large surface area to volume ratio of children permits the rapid cooling and protection of vital organs.)

Craft, Upton. *Key Topics in Anaesthesia*. Bios Scientific Publishers.

A 59. A. false **B.** false **C.** false **D.** false **E.** false

The Glasgow Coma Score (GCS) uses three different aspects of the patient's best responsiveness (eye opening, verbal response and motor response) to provide an assessment of conscious level regardless of the underlying clinical condition or pathological process. Spontaneous eye opening indicates that the arousal mechanisms in the brain stem are active, but does not necessarily imply awareness. This is evaluated by assessing the best verbal response. Motor response reflects the functional state of the brain. The best score from any limb is recorded, even when a difference due to underlying focal cerebral damage exists between the two sides. All painful stimuli should be applied over the patient's fingertips, with pressure applied over the supraorbital notch to test localisation. Extension responses of both upper and lower limbs are always abnormal, whereas a flexion response may on occasion be a normal withdrawal reaction to the applied stimulus. The 'AVPU' system adopts a simple, but more easily remembered, approach to global neurological function in the emergency situation (Awake, Verbalising, Responds to pain, Unresponsive).

Murphy P. *Essays & MCQs in Anaesthesia & Intensive Care*. Edward Arnold, Chapter 15.

A 60. A. true **B.** false **C.** true **D.** false **E.** false

The half-life of COHb is about 250 min when breathing air, 50 min breathing 100% oxygen and 22 min breathing hyperbaric oxygen at 2.4 atmospheres. Haemoglobin partially saturated with carbon monoxide shifts the oxyhaemoglobin dissociation curve to the left. Alkalinisation will move the curve even further to the left and make oxygen delivery worse. Dantrolene reduces increased muscle activity and improves metabolic acidosis. The classical cherry-red appearance is clinically rare. Pulse oximeters over-estimate true percentage oxygen saturation in the presence of COHb but tend towards 85% in the presence of methaemoglobin.

Medicine, Volume 27:4:31.
Hahn CEW, Adams AP. *Pulse Oximetry* by JTB Moyle Series. BMJ Publishing Group, 1994.

Exam 2

Answers

A 1.   **A.** false   **B.** false   **C.** false   **D.** false   **E.** true

Cricoid pressure should be applied over the cricoid cartilage at a force of 10 N at the start of induction and increased to 30 N (3 kg) as the patient loses consciousness. Pressure at this point compresses the oesophagus between the first complete ring of tracheal cartilage and the vertebral body of C6. The seal is improved by leaving a nasogastric tube in place, but it should be gently aspirated first and then left open to air to equalise intragastric pressure with the atmosphere. Preoperative burping may relieve wind from the stomach but in this context the 'backward upward rightward pressure ('BURP')' manoeuvre means re-directing cricoid pressure backwards, upwards and right to improve the view of the larynx at laryngoscopy. It can cause more airway obstruction, so in the event of a failed intubation; cricoid pressure should be applied in the normal fashion. An LMA cannot be correctly placed in the event of a failed intubation while cricoid pressure is applied. Piped medical suction should be capable of generating a vacuum of at least 53 kPa (400 mmHg) and be able to displace at least 40 l/min. An alternative definition states that a unit should take no longer than 10 s to generate a vacuum of 66 kPa (500 mmHg) with a displacement of 25 l/min.

Vanner RG, Asai T. Safe use of cricoid pressure. *Anaesthesia* 1999;54:1–3.

A 2.   **A.** true   **B.** false   **C.** false   **D.** false   **E.** false

Laryngeal mask airways (LMA) may be re-used a limited number of times (usually 40) but require debridement and cleaning as well as sterilisation. Firstly the LMA should be mechanically or manually cleaned both inside and out. The cleaned LMA can then be sterilised by autoclave. Immediately prior to autoclaving, the cuff should be fully deflated. LMAs should be autoclaved in a porous load steam steriliser within a standard cycle at 134°C for 3 min. They should not be exposed to gluteraldehyde, formaldehyde or ethylene oxide. Prolonged immersion in chlorhexidine should be avoided, as these and iodine-based antibiotics and silicon-based lubricant sprays may damage LMAs. Cleansing or wiping with solvent-based solutions and exposure to rinse-aids has a detrimental effect on the silicone compounds and leads to crazing in the polysulfone connector. They should not be subjected to ultrasonic cleansing or γ-irradiation.

A 3. **A.** true **B.** true **C.** false **D.** true **E.** true

Postdural puncture headache has an overall incidence in obstetric practice of 0.5–4%. Incidence following dural puncture with a 16 G Tuohy needle is over 80% but is only 1% following puncture with a pencil-point 25 G spinal needle. Symptoms usually appear 6 h to 2 days later but may occur up to 72 h after puncture. Neck stiffness is common, together with a postural fronto-occipital headache and photophobia. Recognised treatments include epidural infusion of saline, hydration, simple analgesics, oral caffeine and blood patching with >15 ml autologous blood. Initially blood patching was thought to be over 90% successful but recent results suggest that the long-term success rate is as low as 50%. Prophylactic patching is less effective than blood patch delayed until symptoms appear. Abdominal compression transiently relieves the headache making it a useful diagnostic test.

Reynolds F. Dural puncture and headache. *BMJ* 1993;306:874–876.
Turnbull DK, Shepherd DB. Post-dural puncture headache: pathogenesis, prevention and treatment. *BJA* 2003;91:718–729.

A 4. **A.** true **B.** false **C.** false **D.** false **E.** true

These are common drugs that you probably use almost every day. You should know how they are presented. Of the relaxants, suxamethonium and mivacurium are the only chlorides. All the … curoniums are bromides, and … atracuriums are besylates. Gallamine triethiodide is the odd one out. Although fentanyl is a citrate, alfentanil and remifentanil are presented as hydrochlorides. Neostigmine is a methylsulphate, atropine is a sulphate, glycopyrronium is a bromide. All the amide local anaesthetics are hydrochlorides, as is ketamine and most of the inotropes. However, noradrenaline and adrenaline are acid tartrates.

British National Formulary.

A 5. **A.** false **B.** true **C.** false **D.** false **E.** true

Soda lime is made up of calcium hydroxide (94%), sodium hydroxide (5%), potassium hydroxide (1%) and silicates (<1%) for binding. CO_2 in solution reacts with sodium and potassium hydroxides to form carbonates, which then react with calcium hydroxide to produce calcium carbonate and reform the sodium and potassium hydroxide. Heat is produced during the reaction. Trichloroethylene is decomposed by soda lime (with potential neurological toxicity), whereas isoflurane is not.

Yentis, Hirsch, Smith. *Anaesthesia A to Z.* Butterworth Heinemann, 1993.

A 6. **A.** true **B.** true **C.** false **D.** false **E.** false

The dibucaine number represents the degree of inhibition of plasma cholinesterase by dibucaine. It is used as a test for atypical inherited cholinesterase. A normal dibucaine number is 75–85. Homozygotes for the atypical gene have a dibucaine number of 15–25. Heterozygotes have a dibucaine number of 40–60. Homozygotes for the fluoride resistant gene may have a dibucaine number of 65–75 but still demonstrate prolongation of paralysis to suxamethonium for 1–2 h.

Yentis, Hirsch, Smith. *Anaesthesia A to Z.* Butterworth Heinemann, 1993.

A 7. **A.** false **B.** false **C.** true **D.** false **E.** true

This question is difficult to interpret because it asks for AGGRAVATING factors when you might expect to read 'reduced' or 'lessened by'. Always read each leaf against the original question stem. Arterial $PaCO_2$ is the most important regulator of cerebral blood flow (CBF). However, diseased vessels that have lost the ability to autoregulate do not respond to changes in arterial $PaCO_2$. Consequently, for a given cerebral perfusion pressure, hypoventilation-induced hypercapnia will increase CBF by dilating normal cerebral blood vessels resulting in blood being diverted away from ischaemic areas, where the vessels are already maximally dilated ('intracerebral steal'). Conversely, hyperventilation–induced hypocapnia constricts normal cerebral vasculature and may divert blood to already dilated ischaemic areas ('inverse cerebral steal'). Barbiturates decrease cerebral metabolic rate ($CMRO_2$) and blood flow but preserve the 'coupling' between the two and the autoregulatory mechanisms of the cerebral circulation. Used individually or together, both thiopentone and hypothermia have been shown to beneficially reduce $CMRO_2$ in those patients where inadequate cerebral perfusion has been demonstrated but insertion of a shunt is not technically feasible. Other methods shown to be of value in providing pharmacological protection include naloxone, benzodiazepines, etomidate and dextran. In contrast, ketamine causes a direct increase in cerebral metabolism and blood flow as well as pronounced cerebral vasodilatation (i.e. increases $CMRO_2$). Dextrose-containing solutions should be avoided as hyperglycaemia around the time of ischaemia has been shown to be associated with an adverse neurological outcome.

Murphy P. *Essays & MCQs in Anaesthesia and Intensive Care*. Edward Arnold, Chapter 7.

A 8. **A.** false **B.** false **C.** true **D.** false **E.** true

Double-lumen tubes (DLT) allow isolation and independent ventilation of each lung. Although commercially available in right and left forms, left-sided tubes are often preferred. The right upper lobe bronchus, unlike its counterpart on the left, has a variable origin and frequently arises from the main bronchus just beyond the carina (approximately 2 *vs* 5 cm respectively). Placing a right-sided tube accurately is therefore difficult and if done incorrectly or if the tube subsequently becomes dislodged may predispose to hypoxaemia and lobar collapse. To reduce this risk, most right-sided tubes have a ventilation slot built into, or distal, to the bronchial cuff to facilitate right upper lobe ventilation. Left-sided tubes do not need this feature due to the longer left main bronchus. With the exception of surgery involving the left main bronchus, a left-sided tube can be used for any operation on the left lung. Indications for endobronchial intubation (i.e. DLT) range from absolute to relative and include: lung empyema/abscess drainage, bronchopleural fistula closure, major airway trauma, lung and lung cyst resection, video-assisted thoracoscopic surgery, massive intrapulmonary haemorrhage and thoracic aorta/spine and oesophageal surgery. The disposable PVC double-lumen tubes (Bronchocaths) commonly used today are based on the design for a re-usable red rubber DLT originally developed by the British anaesthetist Robertshaw in 1965. Carlens (left-sided) and White (right-sided) endobronchial tubes are even older. Unlike their larger successor, the Robertshaw tube, both possessed a carinal hook to aid positioning.

Gothard, Kelleher. *Essentials of Cardiac and Thoracic Anaesthesia*. Butterworth Heinemann. Chapter 7.

A 9. **A.** true **B.** true **C.** true **D.** false **E.** false

In the classic case of malignant hyperthermia (MH) tachycardia and tachypnoea result from sympathetic nervous system stimulation from hypermetabolism and hypercarbia. Paralysed patients will not exhibit tachypnoea! Hypertension results from sympathetic stimulation and catecholamine release. Suxamethonium may not always trigger MH in an MH-susceptible patient. A potent inhalational agent is sometimes necessary. It has been shown that suxamethonium increases jaw muscle tone in all patients causing masseter muscle rigidity in some. Calcium channel blockers should not be used acutely in MH especially with dantrolene as the combination induces hyperkalaemia. Studies indicate that doses of neuromuscular-blocking agents should not be reduced with dantrolene. The site of action of the former is the nicotinic receptor at the neuromuscular junction and the latter operates within the cell, decreasing intracellular calcium. Dantrolene is a specific agent in MH.

Barash, Cullen, Stoelting. *Clinical Anaesthesia*. Chapter 23.

A 10. **A.** false **B.** false **C.** true **D.** true **E.** true

In patients with end-stage renal disease, suxamethonium is not contraindicated providing the potassium levels are normalised by dialysis. Most uraemic patients will have haemoglobin levels in the range of 6–8 g/dl. If this is chronic, compensatory changes will have occurred that promote oxygen offloading. On this basis transfusion is not mandatory. However, it has been shown to improve allograft survival, perhaps by inducing a degree of specific immunological non-reactivity to the transfused histocompatibility antigens. The response to vecuronium is variable in renal failure. It may accumulate, even post-transplant, as renal metabolic function does not always recover immediately. There are several contraindications to viscera transplantation. These include incurable malignancy, active or incurable systemic infection, old age (physiological), current alcohol or drug abuse, significant obesity and lack of emotional stability or supportive social milieu. In adults the kidney is transplanted retroperitoneally. Revascularisation of the allograft involves anastomosing the renal vessels to an iliac artery and vein. This necessitates clamping the common iliac vessels resulting in lower limb ischaemia. On release, renal preservative solution and venous drainage (both rich in potassium) enter the circulation.

Barash, Cullen, Stoelting. *Clinical Anaesthesia*, 2nd Edn. Chapter 55.

A 11. A. false **B.** false **C.** true **D.** false **E.** true

As far as day case surgery is concerned, age limits are controversial. Usually children under one are excluded but minor procedures may be performed under this age if patients were not born prematurely. Babies under six months should be excluded. Patients over 70 years are usually excluded. Surgery should not be expected to take longer than one hour! However, many units bend this rule by judicious organisation of the list order to allow a longer period of recovery. Epidurals and spinals have been performed but in the UK it is uncommon. Patients must be ASA I or II though well–controlled diabetics or hypertensives may be included for minor procedures. Patients must be accompanied home by an able person and have access to a telephone easily.

Yentis, Hirsch, Smith. *Anaesthesia A to Z.* Butterworth Heinemann.

A 12. A. true **B.** false **C.** true **D.** false **E.** true

Magnetic resonance imaging (MRI) requires the patient to be inserted into a powerful magnetic field. Nuclei with an odd number of protons or neutrons such as sodium, hydrogen, phosphorus and carbon respond to the magnetic resonance. The magnets are energised constantly, so precautions need to be taken at all times, e.g. removing all metal objects, wristwatches, credit cards from personal effects before entry. Whilst the magnetic field is thought to be safe (so the anaesthetist can be present at all times), the anaesthetic machine and monitors may need to be remote from the patient (at least 3 m away to the side, or 5 m away front to back.) Anaesthetic machines and monitors without ferromagnetic material have been described. Modern cerebral vascular aneurysm clips are MRI compatible but artificial pacemakers are not.

Nimmo, Rowbotham, Smith. *Anaesthesia*, 2nd Edn. Blackwell Scientific Publications, Chapter 41.

A 13. A. true **B.** true **C.** true **D.** true **E.** true

Acute haemolytic reactions due to transfusion incompatibility present with fever, nausea, shaking and pain in the flank and chest. Febrile reactions (a rise of more than 1°C) are the most common complication of blood transfusion. They can be avoided by using white-cell-depleted saline-washed red cells or microaggregate filters. Febrile reactions are relatively benign. Recognition of a haemolytic reaction may be difficult during anaesthesia and the appearance of red urine due to haemolysis or DIC could be the first sign. Allergic reactions are the second most common reaction of transfusion and may manifest with hives. Delayed haemolytic reaction may occur in patients having received compatible cross-matched blood over a 4- to 21-day period, due to red cell destruction. It is usually subclinical and diagnosed by a positive Coomb's test.

Barash, Cullen, Stoelting. *Clinical Anaesthesia*, 2nd Edn. Chapter 11.

A 14. A. true **B.** true **C.** true **D.** true **E.** true

Complications of retrobulbar block may be systemic or local. Retrobulbar blockade requires the injection of local anaesthetic into the muscle cone behind the eye. The most common complication is retrobulbar haemorrhage due to puncturing of the vessels within the retrobulbar space. The increased pressure in the globe can cause central artery occlusion. Other complications include bradycardia secondary to the oculocardiac reflex, posterior globe puncture with resultant retinal detachment and vitreous haemorrhage, penetration of the optic nerve, brain stem anaesthesia from local entering breeched dura around the optic nerve and subarachnoid blockade or inadvertent intraocular or intravascular injection; hence, the preference of most anaesthetists for peribulbar blocks.

Barash, Cullen, Stoelting. *Clincal Anaesthesia*, 2nd Edn. Chapter 38.

A **15.** **A.** false   **B.** true   **C.** false   **D.** false   **E.** true

A recovery area was first described by Florence Nightingale in 1863 but first opened in the USA in 1923. The first in the UK was in 1955. It is sufficient to have 1.5 bays per theatre with one to one nursing, until the patient is able to maintain their own airway.

Yentis, Hirsch, Smith. *Anaesthesia A to Z*. Butterworth Heinemann.

A **16.** **A.** true   **B.** false   **C.** false   **D.** false   **E.** false

The brachial plexus can be approached from above or below during regional anaesthesia for surgery on the upper arm. The interscalene approach gives excellent anaesthesia to the shoulder and upper arm, but commonly leads to inadequate blockade of the ulnar nerve. Potential side effects of this block are Horner's syndrome, phrenic nerve block, recurrent laryngeal nerve block and inadvertent extradural or intrathecal injection. Bilateral interscalene blocks should not be performed. The supraclavicular approach commonly leads to inadequate blockade of the median nerve. Horner's syndrome and pneumothorax are amongst the adverse events that can occur with this approach. The axillary approach commonly leads to inadequate blockade of the axillary nerve, and supplemental subcutaneous local anaesthetic will be required if the upper/outer aspect of the arm is involved in surgery, or if a tourniquet is to be used. Horner's syndrome does not occur with the axillary approach.

Yentis, Hirsch, Smith. *Anaesthesia A to Z*. Butterworth Heinemann, 1993.

A **17.** **A.** true   **B.** true   **C.** true   **D.** true   **E.** true

Vagotonic drugs and stimuli, β-blockade plus or minus calcium channel blockade have all been shown to increase the likelihood of bradycardia in association with high plasma concentrations of opioids. Peak plasma concentration of remifentanil is reduced by administration as a slow intravenous injection over a period of more than 30 s.

Miller. *Anaesthesia*, 4th Edn.

A **18.** **A.** true **B.** true **C.** false **D.** true **E.** true

Rocuronium bromide (Esmeron) is presented as a liquid (10 mg/ml solution) containing sodium acetate, sodium chloride and acetic acid. It is known to be incompatible with barbiturates, numerous antibiotics, steroids, frusemide, and others. The ED90 (dose required to produce 90% depression of the twitch response of the thumb to stimulation of the ulnar nerve) during balanced anaesthesia is approximately 0.3 mg/kg body weight. Recommended intubating dose is 0.6 mg/kg, although this can be increased to 1.0 mg/kg as part of a rapid sequence induction. Doses over 0.9 mg/kg may increase heart rate. 30% of the total administered dose is recoverable from the urine in the first 12 h postoperatively. No plasma or urine metabolites have been detected. Hepatic excretion probably occurs too. In animal studies 30–40% was excreted unchanged in bile.

Esmeron Data Sheet.

A **19.** **A.** false **B.** true **C.** true **D.** false **E.** true

Sevoflurane has been shown to degrade to Compound A upon interaction with carbon dioxide absorbents. Compound A is more correctly termed fluoromethyl-2,2-difluoro-1-(trifluoromethyl)vinyl ether. During sevoflurane anaesthesia, factors that increase Compound A concentration include use of low-flow or closed-circuit anaesthesia, the use of baralyme rather than soda lime, higher concentrations of sevoflurane in the circuit, higher absorbent temperatures and fresh absorbent. It is said that the degradation products do not cause clinically detectable toxic effects in humans even during low-flow anaesthesia. In the presence of alkali and heat, trichloroethylene is also degraded by soda lime, but into the cranial neurotoxin dichloroacetylene. Phosgene, a potent pulmonary irritant, is also produced resulting in cranial nerve lesions, encephalitis and ARDS.

Miller. *Anaesthesia*, 4th Edn. Chapter 9.

A 20. **A.** true **B.** false **C.** false **D.** true **E.** true

Xenon is a very dense gas that is non-explosive and non-irritant. It has a MAC of 71% (N_2O has a MAC of 104%). Its blood-gas solubility is 0.085 compared with N_2O at 0.47 making the potential for alterations in depth of anaesthesia even more rapid. Anaesthesia is very cardiostable ... but very expensive.

Barash, Cullen, Stoetling. *Handbook of Clinical Anaesthesia*, 2nd Edn. Lippincott.

A 21. **A.** true **B.** true **C.** true **D.** false **E.** false

The intrinsic capacity of a ventricular muscle strip to contract in response to 'preload' (a weight distending the resting strip) and in the face of 'afterload' (a second weight only imposed during contraction) is affected by its contractility. Measuring myocardial contractility *in vivo* is complicated and requires that end diastolic volume ('preload'), the forces opposing ventricular contraction ('afterload') and heart rate (that may by itself affect contractility) are kept constant. Although dP/dtmax has been used as a measure of myocardial contractility, the forces opposing myocardial contraction change during ejection due to the flow of blood and the elastic properties of the arterial tree. The left ventricular end systolic pressure-volume relationship avoids intrasystolic complexity and is preload independent but non-linear during ischaemia. Inotropic agents normally enhance systolic contraction and diastolic relaxation (lusitropy). Dopexamine is not a direct agonist at cardiac β_1 receptors that are normally responsible for chronotropy and contractility but can increase contractility because of noradrenaline reuptake inhibition.

A 22. **A.** true **B.** false **C.** false **D.** true **E.** false

Nitric oxide causes a rise in cyclic guanosine monophosphate in smooth muscle cells. Nitric oxide is a poor bronchodilator but may enhance other efficient bronchodilators. NADH- or NADPH-dependent methaemoglobin reductases are the main enzymes responsible for reconverting the ferric iron of haemoglobin back to its normal ferrous state. These systems can be overwhelmed when nitric oxide is used pharmacologically. Nitric oxide can only be mixed with oxygen just prior to administration because it is

converted within minutes to nitrous oxide and nitrous acid
(if water is present), which damages the lung.

Tibballs J in *Paediatric Intensive Care*. Duncan A (ed). BMJ Publishing
Group, 1998.

A 23. **A.** false **B.** false **C.** false **D.** true **E.** true

Acid-secreting parietal cells and pepsinogen-secreting chief cells
are found in the upper two thirds of the stomach.

Kumar, Clark. *Clinical Medicine*, 3rd Edn. Saunders, Chapter 4.

A 24. **A.** true **B.** true **C.** false **D.** true **E.** true

Pulmonary vascular resistance can be measured in mmHg/l/min or
dynes.sec.cm^{-5}. A dyne is a unit of force which, when acting on a
mass of 1 g will cause it to accelerate at 1 cm/s^{-1}. In the lateral
decubitus position blood flow is relatively gravity dependent.
The degree of ventilation depends on the state of the patient.
The lower diaphragm tends to be opposed by the weight of the
abdominal contents, but contracts well with spontaneous
ventilation. However, in an anaesthetised and paralysed patient,
the dependent lung is overperfused (gravity) and
underventilated (diaphragm splinting and mediastinal weight).
The situation is more marked when the chest is opened,
removing the restrictive effect of the chest wall. However,
remember that this is only true for positive pressure ventilation
since the resultant pneumothorax would decrease spontaneous
ventilation of the open side of the chest.

Prys-Roberts, Brown. *International Practice of Anaesthesia*. Butterworth
Heinemann, Chapters 56 and 59.
Barash, Cullen, Stoelting. *Handbook of Clinical Anaesthesia*. Lippincott,
Chapter 6.

A 25. **A.** true **B.** true **C.** true **D.** true **E.** false

The International Association for the Study of Pain (IASP) defines
hyperalgesia as an increased response to a stimulus which is
normally painful. The IASP definition of allodynia is pain due to a
stimulus which does not normally evoke pain. Both A delta and C

fibre nociceptors progressively lower their excitation threshold in response to repeated noxious stimuli.

Prys-Roberts, Brown. *International Practice of Anaesthesia*. Butterworth Heinemann, Chapter 2.

A **26.** **A.** false   **B.** true   **C.** false   **D.** false   **E.** true

Radiofrequency ablation relies on an alternating current flowing through tissue from one small electrode to an appropriately placed secondary electrode usually a large flat plate. However, it is the molecular movement induced in the tissue by the electromagnetic field produced rather than the current that produces the heat. Lesions are produced at 45°C and a thermocouple on the probe senses this. Lesions are usually 1 mm deep with a diameter of 5 mm but relies on tissue homogeneity for the expected shape.

Cosman E *et al*. Theoretical aspects of radiofrequency lesions in the dorsal root entry zone. *Neurosurgery* 1984;15:945–950.

A **27.** **A.** true   **B.** false   **C.** false   **D.** true   **E.** true

WHO ECG diagnostic criteria for MI include >1 mm ST elevation in the standard leads or ≥2 mm ST elevation in adjacent chest leads. The angiographic limb of the GUSTO-II trial showed that ST elevation reflected acute coronary occlusion in 87% of cases. TIMI 3 flow as defined in the question is thought necessary for effective thrombolysis but only occurs in around 50%. 30% of early patent arteries are re-occluded by between 3 and 6 months.

Acute Coronary Syndromes. *Lancet* 1999;353(suppl II):1–26.
Swanton R. *Cardiology*. Blackwell Science, 1998.
Howell S *et al*. *Br J Anaesth* 1998;80:14–19.

A **28.** **A.** true   **B.** false   **C.** false   **D.** false   **E.** true

MG was first described by Willis in 1672. 90% of patients with MG and thymoma have antistriated muscle antibodies. High dose and rapid introduction of high-dose corticosteroids is associated with exacerbations, myasthenic crises, myopathy and the need for postoperative ventilation. In severely ill patients acute high-dose steroids might be justified to obtain a quick response but plasma exchange or intravenous immunoglobulin could obtain a rapid effect without these risks if necessary preoperatively. The IV equivalent of anticholinesterases is 30 times smaller than the oral dose. MG is not normally improved by removal of a thymoma which although usually benign may cause local effects. Thymectomy for thymic hyperplasia is effective in about 85% of cases but in general the improvement is noted 1–10 years postoperatively. Surgery itself may aggravate MG. The usual dose of pyridostigmine is 30–120 mg 3–4 hourly, except at night. High doses increase the risk of cholinergic crisis and postoperative ventilation. Other risk factors include MG for more than 6 years, a history of chronic respiratory disease and a preoperative vital capacity of less than 2.9 L.

Baraka A. *Can J Anaesth* 1992;39:476.
Drachman D. *N Engl J Med* 1994;330:1797–1810.
Newsom-Davis J. *Medicine* 1996;24(6):110–113.

A 29. **A.** false   **B.** false   **C.** true   **D.** false   **E.** true

In Duchenne muscular dystrophy there is muscle degeneration with normal innervation. Inheritance is X-linked recessive. It is the most severe and most common of the muscular dystrophies, commencing in males between 2 and 5 years of age and typically affecting proximal muscles especially the pelvis. Most are unable to walk by 10 years and die of pneumonia often by 20 years. Restrictive ventilatory defects are common from kyphoscoliosis. Cardiomyopathies are common with arrhythmias and a decreased ventricular contractility. There is no definite response to muscle relaxants but non-depolarising agents may have a prolonged recovery time and response to suxamethonium may be abnormal.

Nimmo, Rowbotham, Smith. *Anaesthesia*, 2nd Edn, Volume 2.

A 30. **A.** false   **B.** false   **C.** false   **D.** false   **E.** false

Myasthenic syndrome complicates around 1% of bronchogenic carcinomas and older males are the most commonly affected. Diagnosis may pre-date the diagnosis of a malignancy by several years. Proximal muscles of the lower limb are most commonly affected and bulbar muscle involvement is rare. Muscle strength improves with exercise, and tetanic stimulation results in a progressive increase in twitch height. Anticholinesterases have no effect. There is sensitivity to suxamethonium and non-depolarising agents, unlike with myasthenia gravis.

Nimmo, Rowbotham, Smith. *Anaesthesia*, 2nd Edn, Volume 2.

A 31. A. false **B.** true **C.** true **D.** true **E.** true

CF is the commonest autosomal recessive disease (1 in 2,000). One in 22 Caucasians are carriers. Cystic fibrosis is due to an abnormality in the cystic fibrosis transmembrane conductance regulator (CFTR) encoded on chromosome 7, which is probably a chloride channel. This causes decreased excretion of chloride into the airway secretions, resulting in increased reabsorption of sodium and water and increased viscosity of the secretions. Sweat Na^+ is GREATER than 60 mmol/l. Chloride secretion by the sweat glands is independent of the CFTR.

Collier, Longmore, Hodgetts. *Oxford Handbook of Clinical Specialties*, 4th Edn. OUP, p 192.

A 32. A. false **B.** false **C.** true **D.** true **E.** true

Acute liver failure (ALF) is defined by the occurrence of encephalopathy, coagulopathy and jaundice in an individual with a previously normal liver. Worldwide it is caused mainly by hepatotrophic viruses (A–E) but in the UK the most common cause is paracetamol overdose. Cardiovascular changes in ALF are similar to septic shock with hypotension, low SVR and high cardiac output. Oliguric renal failure is common, occurring in up to 75% of cases caused by paracetamol overdose and 30–50% of others.

Management of acute liver failure. Lai WK, Murphy N. *Continuing Education in Anaesthesia, Critical Care & Pain.* BJA publications, Volume 4, Number 2, April 2004.

A 33. A. true **B.** true **C.** true **D.** false **E.** true

Axial involvement in rheumatoid arthritis probably occurs in more than 80% of cases. Atlantoaxial subluxation, a feared complication risking cord compression during positioning for intubation, occurs in approximately 25% and may be entirely asymptomatic. A distance on lateral X-ray of >3 mm between the peg and the atlas in patients less than 44 years and >4 mm if older than 44 years is an indicator of joint disruption. However, there is space in the vertebral canal at this point that may protect the cord under normal everyday circumstances and 8 mm of odontoid separation is much more likely to be associated with cord compression. Airflow obstruction occurs in 30%. A restrictive defect may also occur in the form of fibrosing alveolitis or methotrexate therapy.

Wordsworth B in *Rheumatoid Arthritis in Oxford Textbook of Medicine*, 3rd Edn. Weatherall D, Ledingham J, Warrell D (eds). Oxford University Press, 1996.

A **34.** **A.** true **B.** false **C.** false **D.** true **E.** false

It is very rare for clotting to become significantly deranged without coexistent thrombocytopaenia. In most studies of severe pre-eclampsia there is a poor correlation between left- and right-sided cardiac filling pressure measurements. This data is used to support monitoring with pulmonary artery flotation catheters, although the effect on outcome is unproven. Magnesium sulphate 40 mg/kg on induction has been shown to be at least, if not more, effective than alfentanil at controlling the pressor response to intubation in pre-eclampsia. ACEIs are contraindicated throughout pregnancy. In early pregnancy they are associated with oligohydramnios and possibly skull malformation, and at term they are a cause of neonatal hypotension and oligo- or anuria.

Gatt S in *Baillieres Clinical Obstetrics and Gynaecology*. Arulkumaran S (ed) 1999;13(1):95–105.
British Medical Bulletin.

A **35.** **A.** false **B.** true **C.** false **D.** true **E.** false

The lack of correlation of site of MI and coronary disease may in part explain why prophylactic angioplasty prior to surgery remains an unproven method of improving perioperative outcome. GTN requires enzymatic conversion to nitric oxide (unlike nitroprusside) and is less effective when sulphur-hydryl groups have been consumed. The major risk for hypotension on induction appears to be for patients taking ACEIs for hypertension. Physiologically these patients are more likely to have lower blood volumes after inhibition of aldosterone release. The current American and European consensus is that prophylactic CABG does not benefit patients with coronary disease requiring non-coronary surgery unless the patient would benefit from CABG for accepted indications as well.

Metzler H, Fleischer L, Coriat P, Gouille L in *Baillieres Clinical Anaesthesiology* 12:3. List W, Metzler H (eds). 1998, pp 419–432 and 405–418 respectively.
Transiderm-Nitro Trial Study Group. *J Am Coll Cardiology* 1989;13:786–793.
Prospective randomised study of intensive insulin treatment on long term survival after acute MI in patients with diabetes mellitus. DIGAMI study group. *BMJ* 314(24);1512–1515.

A 36. A. false   **B.** false   **C.** false   **D.** false   **E.** true

Following heart-lung transplants patients have no cough reflex from below the tracheal anastomosis. Cardiac or trans-bronchial biopsies are used to investigate rejection. Resting heart rate is high due to lack of vagal tone on the SA node. Coronary flow is increased due to denervation of α-receptors.

Prys-Roberts, Brown. *International Practice of Anaesthesia*, 1st Edn. Butterworth Heinemann, Chapter 67.

A 37. A. true   **B.** false   **C.** true   **D.** true   **E.** false

Exposure and decortication of bone during scoliosis surgery is usually associated with major blood loss.

Prys-Roberts, Brown. *International Practice of Anaesthesia*. Butterworth Heinemann, Chapter 114.

A 38. A. true   **B.** true   **C.** false   **D.** true   **E.** true

The important five diseases presenting with the triad of weight loss, anaemia and slight lemon yellow tinge are: carcinoma of the stomach, carcinoma of the caecum, carcinoma of the pancreas, pernicious anaemia and uraemia.

Ellis, Calne. *Lecture Notes in General Surgery*. Blackwell, Chapter 22.

A 39. A. false   **B.** false   **C.** false   **D.** true   **E.** false

The most common intraocular surgical procedure is cataract extraction. This is now predominantly undertaken under local anaesthesia. The eyelid is held open by levator palpebrae superioris supplied by the oculomotor and sympathetic nerves. Blockade of the seventh nerve supplying orbicularis oculi aids surgery by preventing blinking. Although the oculocardiac reflex can be ablated by an established block, one of the complications of block insertion is provocation of this reflex. Amaurosis is an uncommon feature of peribulbar block because the optic nerve is inside the 'cone' of extraocular muscles, and therefore it is more likely to be a feature of retrobulbar injection of local anaesthetic.

Eke T *et al*. The National Survey of Local Anaesthesia for Ocular Surgery I. Survey methodology and current practice. *Eye* 1999;13(Pt 2):189–195.
Johnson R. Anatomy for ophthalmic anaesthesia. *Br J Anaesth* 1995;75:80–87.
Rubin A. Complications of local anaesthesia for ophthalmic surgery. *Br J Anaesth* 1995;75:93–96.

[A] 40. **A.** true   **B.** false   **C.** true   **D.** false   **E.** false

Octreotide, a somatostatin analogue has been used to try and reduce pancreatic enzyme production. The Ranson criteria are not diagnostic. They are used to indicate prognosis and stratify illness severity but do not require measurement of amylase. CT scanning is indicated for a Ranson score >3, patients not improving after 72 h and patients who deteriorate after initial improvement. An enlarged pancreas with more than two fluid collections predicts a >50% chance of developing an abscess requiring drainage. Ampicillin has poor pancreatic penetration. Carbapenems are more appropriate. Surgical intervention in pancreatitis is controversial. However, two studies have suggested that in severe gallstone pancreatitis early sphincterotomy and stone extraction reduces morbidity.

Coad N. Acute severe pancreatitis. *Br J Intens Care* 1999;9:38–45.

[A] 41. **A.** false   **B.** true   **C.** true   **D.** false   **E.** false

When normally saturated, modern pulse oximeters have a mean error of <2%. However, accuracy falls significantly below saturations of 80%. The presence of methaemoglobin causes oximeters to tend to 85%. The venous pulsation seen in patients with severe tricuspid incompetence is misinterpreted as arterial pulsation and can lead to falsely low readings. Intravenous methylene blue administration causes a transient falsely low reading. Jaundice has no effect on oximetry readings *in vivo*.

Nimmo, Rowbotham, Smith. *Anaesthesia*, 2nd Edn. Blackwell Scientific Publications, Chapter 35.

A **42.** **A.** false **B.** true **C.** false **D.** true **E.** true

Whilst the presence of carbon dioxide in the expired gas is an important sign after intubation, significant quantities of carbon dioxide can be present in the stomach, and detection of carbon dioxide in the first few breaths may not exclude oesophageal intubation. Sudden falls in end-tidal carbon dioxide concentrations may be caused by acute circulatory failure. Increases will occur with malignant hyperthermia, developing fever, respiratory centre depression, reduced ventilation or acute respiratory distress. Mainstream analysers, because of their bulk and weight, may contribute to 'disconnect' incidents by dragging on the endotracheal tube/catheter mount connection. Sidestream analysers aspirate up to 150 ml of gas/min, thus creating a significant 'leak' if low flow anaesthesia is being utilised. Some systems allow the analysed exhaust gas to be returned to the breathing system thus eliminating this problem.

Nimmo, Rowbotham, Smith. *Anaesthesia*, 2nd Edn. Blackwell Scientific Publications, Chapter 35.

A **43.** **A.** false **B.** true **C.** true **D.** true **E.** true

The forced vital capacity (FVC) is commonly reduced in both obstructive and restrictive lung disease; however, a reduction of the forced expiratory volume in 1 s (FEV$_1$) to FVC ratio below 0.7 represents obstructive airway disease. All respiratory function tests vary with age, height and sex. Maximum expiratory flow-volume curves have characteristic shapes for normal airways, large airway obstruction and small airway obstruction. FVC is reduced by 50% following major abdominal surgery.

Nimmo, Rowbotham, Smith. *Anaesthesia*, 2nd Edn. Blackwell Scientific Publications. Chapter 35.

A **44.** **A.** true   **B.** true   **C.** true   **D.** true   **E.** true

Trans-oesophageal echocardiography (TOE) provides anatomical and physiological information about the heart and great vessels. It can be used intraoperatively to measure changes in ventricular cavity size during the cardiac cycle and derive end-systolic/diastolic volumes and, consequently, ventricular ejection fraction. The addition of Doppler colour flow imaging provides information about the direction and velocity of blood flow. This flow imaging technology can be used intraoperatively to demonstrate and quantify any valvular dysfunction. Myocardial wall motion is a sensitive marker of myocardial perfusion and the development of regional wall motion abnormalities (RWMA) is likely to represent myocardial ischaemia. However, it should be appreciated that RWMA may be caused by factors other than ischaemia such as 'stunned' myocardium, previous myocardial infarction, hypothermia and changes in ventricular loading. TOE is a useful diagnostic technique in thoracic aortic dissection for demonstrating the true and false lumina. It has also been used to detect intracardiac air emboli during certain open neurosurgical procedures and is frequently used by cardiac surgeons to assess the adequacy of valvular and septal repairs prior to the closure of the chest.

Goldhill, Strunin. *Clinical Anaesthesiology: The High-risk Surgical Patient.* Bailliere, Chapter 1.
Murphy P. *Essays & MCQs in Anaesthesia and Intensive Care.* Edward Arnold, Chapter 5.

A **45.** **A.** true   **B.** true   **C.** true   **D.** false   **E.** false

There are many devices available for measuring volume and flow. The vitalograph has a motor-driven chart and bellows. The Benedict Roth spirometer involves a bell and rotating drum. The Bourdon gauge is a fixed orifice device. The vitalograph and Benedict Roth spirometers are used for measuring volumes of up to a few litres. The vitalograph is more portable than the Benedict Roth spirometer. The dry gas meter is better for measuring large volumes.

Parbrook GD, Davis PD, Parbrook EO. *Basic Physics and Measurement in Anaesthesia.* Heinnemann.

Humidification of gases can be achieved in a variety of ways. The simple water bath relies on bubbling dry gases through water at room temperature. Efficiency can be increased by reducing bubble size with sintered glass. Latent heat of vaporisation is a problem with the water bath and can be reduced by adding an electric heater. Hot element humidifiers are unsuitable for use with volatile agents because the heat can cause chemical changes. The ideal size of droplets produced by nebulisers is 1 μm. Droplets over 20 μm may form pools of water in tubing. Small droplets are stable, carry for long distances and may be a source of cross-infection.

Parbrook GD, Davis PD, Parbrook EO. *Basic Physics and Measurement in Anaesthesia*. Heinnemann.

A 47. **A.** false **B.** false **C.** false **D.** true **E.** false

A low CVP is likely to be found in both hypovolaemic and septic shock as both conditions require filling with fluid in the first instance. A raised SVR is consistent with both hypovolaemic and cardiogenic shock. The cardiac output may initially rise in hypovolaemic shock but will fall back as the state is allowed to continue and the myocardium becomes more ischaemic. Since nitric-oxide-induced vasodilatation does not occur in hypovolaemia, there is no role for a nitric oxide inhibitor.

Oh T. *Intensive Care Manual*, 4th Edn. Butterworth Heinemann, Chapters 14 and 15.

A 48. **A.** false **B.** true **C.** false **D.** false **E.** true

α-adrenergic effects are mediated through an inositol phosphate pathway (not cyclic adenosine monophosphate). Dopexamine is an ino-dilator and the phosphodiesterase inhibitors should not be used in severe heart failure because there appears to be an increased mortality associated with their use in these patients. Digoxin has minimal effects as an inotrope and potential for toxicity is increased by hypokalaemia, hypomagnesaemia, hypercalcaemia, hypoxia and acidosis.

Oh T. *Intensive Care Manual*, 4th Edn. Butterworth Heinemann, Chapter 12.

Exam 3

Answers

A **49.** **A.** false **B.** true **C.** true **D.** false **E.** true

1,500 people die from asthma each year in the UK. Standard treatment of acute severe asthma includes sitting the patient up, high flow oxygen, bronchodilators (β_2-agonists and anticholinergics) given by nebuliser or intravenously, and anti-inflammatory drugs e.g. corticosteroids. Fall-back therapy has in the past included the use of ketamine and bronchodilator inhalational anaesthetic agents. Recent guidelines suggest the use of a single IV dose of magnesium sulphate in life-threatening asthma in patients who have not had a good initial response to inhaled bronchodilator therapy. The guideline does not recommend the magnesium for use in children aged 2–5 years. Recommended adult dose range is 1.2–2 g (4.8–8 mmol) which equates to 2.4–4 ml of a 50% solution. Magnesium works by relaxing bronchial smooth muscle, inhibiting acetylcholine release at the neuromuscular junction and stabilising mast cells. The recommended dose produces a fall in blood pressure of about 5 mmHg and causes burning at the IV injection site, flushing and fatigue in over half of patients.

Drugs and Therapeutics Bulletin, Volume 41, Number 10, October 2003. British Thoracic Society Guidelines 2003.

A **50.** **A.** true **B.** false **C.** false **D.** true **E.** true

Anaphylaxis is an IgE-mediated type 1 hypersensitivity reaction resulting in widespread mast cell degranulation and basophil activation in response to a specific allergen. Cardiovascular collapse is the most common physical sign occurring in 90% of patients, with bronchospasm being present in 50%. Elevation of C3 and C4 complement levels indicate an immune-mediated response while elevation of C3 alone suggests alternative pathway activation.

Craft TM, Nolan JP, Parr MJA. *Key topics in Critical Care*, 1st Edn. BIOS Scientific Publishers Ltd.

A **51.** **A.** true **B.** true **C.** true **D.** false **E.** true

Lamotrigene is one of the newer antiepilepsy drugs used as a second- or third-line treatment in chronic epilepsy, but not in status.

Oh T. *Intensive Care Manual*, 4th Edn. Butterworth Heinemann, Chapter 41.

A 52. **A.** true   **B.** false   **C.** false   **D.** true   **E.** true

Hyperosmolar non-ketotic coma is much less common than diabetic ketoacidosis. About 30% are previously undiagnosed diabetics. The prodromal illness may be lengthy (weeks) and mortality is high (40–70%). Coma may be precipitated by steroid administration but not by antibiotic administration. Severe dehydration occurs and serum osmolality is high.

Oh T. *Intensive Care Manual*. Butterworth, 4th Edn. 1997, Chapter 50.

A 53. **A.** false   **B.** false   **C.** true   **D.** true   **E.** false

Neurogenic diabetes insipidus is caused by a lack of antidiuretic hormone and is also seen after severe head injury. Nephrogenic diabetes insipidus is caused by renal tubular resistance to antidiuretic hormone. A number of drugs can cause nephrogenic diabetes insipidus including frusemide, lithium, gentamicin and glibenclamide. It is also seen in hypercalcaemia and hypokalaemia.

Oh T. *Intensive Care Manual*. Butterworth, 4th Edn. 1997.

A 54. **A.** false   **B.** false   **C.** false   **D.** false   **E.** false

Fat embolism syndrome usually presents 24–72 h following the initial insult. Classically pulmonary, cutaneous and cerebral manifestations are found. Headache and irritability are common cerebral manifestations with coma and convulsions occurring in severe cases. The petechial rash develops in non-dependent areas (classically the chest, axilla, and conjunctiva). Fat in the urine is neither sensitive nor specific enough to aid diagnosis.

Oh T. *Intensive Care Manual*. Butterworth, 4th Edn. 1997, Chapter 31.

A 55. **A.** false   **B.** true   **C.** false   **D.** false   **E.** false

The GCS score ranges from 3 to 15 and was developed for head-injured patients. It is split into three assessment areas: eye opening (1–4), best verbal response (1–5), and best motor response (1–6). Paediatric versions are available for small children. A score of 8 or below represents coma. The Glasgow outcome score defines five levels of possible outcome.

Oh T. *Intensive Care Manual*. Butterworth, 4th Edn. 1997, Chapter 2.

Answers

A 56. A. false **B.** false **C.** true **D.** true **E.** true

It is important that the anaesthetist is aware of the significance of the various serological markers of Hepatitis B, as anaesthesia and surgery during the acute phase of the illness may be associated with a serious deterioration in liver function. During active infection elective surgery should be postponed for at least 6 months. HBs antigen is the first marker indicating acute infection. It appears from about 6 weeks to 3 months and may then disappear or persist. Its continuing presence beyond 3 months usually indicates chronic, ongoing infection (10–15% of cases) or the development of an asymptomatic carrier state (5% of cases). HBe antigen rises early and usually declines rapidly. It correlates with an increased severity and infectivity of disease. High titres in the blood beyond 3 months suggest the development of chronic liver disease or a high risk of infectivity chronic carrier state. Anti-HBs antibody appears late in the disease and indicates immunity. Anti-HBc (IgM) antibody, in contrast, is the first antibody to appear and persists for many months. Persisting high titres beyond 6 months indicate either ongoing infection or the development of a chronic carrier state. Anti-HBe antibody appears after Anti-HBc antibody. Its persistence in high titres beyond 6 months indicates the persistence of a low risk of infectivity chronic carrier state.

Murphy P. *Essays & MCQs in Anaesthesia and Intensive Care*. Edward Arnold, Chapter 18.

A 57. A. true **B.** true **C.** false **D.** true **E.** true

Although *Escherichia coli* is a normal gut commensal, *E. coli* 0157 is a toxic variant that was first reported as a human pathogen in 1982. Case reports have steadily risen in number from 50 in 1985 to 1,050 in 1995. *E. coli* 0157 multiplies naturally in the intestines of cattle, and has recently been found in sheep. It does not cause animal symptoms. Calves are particularly likely to be *E. coli* 0157 carriers. Human infection is most likely to occur via contamination of ground beef and unpasteurised milk. Paddling pools and lakes have been documented as a source of infection (probably via human or animal diarrhoea in unchlorinated water). Haemolytic uraemic syndrome is the commonest cause of ARF in children in the Western world. The syndrome comprises haemolytic anaemia, low platelet count and renal failure. The commonest form occurs in children and is preceded by a diarrhoeal illness. The majority of cases are associated with verocytotoxin producing *E. coli*. Prognosis is good, mortality being around 3–7%. 15–40% have long-term renal impairment. Other complications include thrombotic thrombocytopaenic purpura with CNS involvement, mainly in adults and associated with a poor prognosis. The Scottish outbreak in 1996 involved 479 reported cases and caused 20 deaths.

H.U.S.H. (Haemolytic Uraemic Syndrome Help). UK *E. coli* support group.

A 58. A. true **B.** true **C.** false **D.** true **E.** false

Following salicylate (aspirin) overdose arterial blood gas analysis usually shows a mixed picture of respiratory alkalosis and metabolic acidosis. Direct stimulation of the respiratory centre results in a compensatory increase in bicarbonate excretion by the kidneys. Accompanying potassium and water excretion then result in hypokalaemia, dehydration and metabolic acidosis. The latter is further exacerbated in severe poisoning by an uncoupling of oxidative phosphorylation and inhibition of the tricarboxylic acid cycle (increased circulating levels of pyruvate and lactate). Non-cardiogenic pulmonary oedema occasionally develops in the presence of a reduced circulating volume due to increased pulmonary vascular permeability. Other clinical features include: sweating, hyperpyrexia, nausea and vomiting, irritability, tinnitus and deafness. In the absence of hypoglycaemia, coma is unusual although there may be drowsiness and stupor. Treatment consists of gastric aspiration and lavage, combined with careful fluid balance and electrolyte replacement. Urinary pH is initially alkaline but then becomes acidic. Forced alkaline diuresis may therefore be of value in encouraging salicylate excretion by altering ionisation but should be used with caution and only used to counter high plasma levels (>750 mg/l).

Murphy P. *Essays & MCQs in Anaesthesia and Intensive Care*. Edward Arnold, Chapter 16.

A 59. A. true **B.** false **C.** false **D.** false **E.** true

In patients with a severe thermal injury, there is an immediate loss of gut mucosal integrity followed by a more delayed depression of cellular immunity. The latter is characterised by impaired phagocyte function and decreased neutrophil chemotaxis; this is aggravated further by the effects of the gut-derived endotoxaemia. Sepsis and multiple organ failure are the leading causes of death in this group of patients. Meticulous nursing care, early excision of infected or devitalised tissue combined with early enteral feeding and wound closure with skin grafting offers the best chance of survival for these patients. Although at a high risk of infection, systemic antibiotics should only be prescribed when a pathogen has been identified either in serial blood cultures or wound biopsies. This helps to prevent the emergence of resistance. Several studies have shown that, in the absence of inhalation injury, there is no significant microvascular permeability defect to protein in the lungs or non-burned tissue. The increase in lung interstitial water and generalised tissue oedema that follows is due to a combination of a hypoproteinaemic state and a mediator-induced inflammatory response. Ambient temperature should ideally be maintained between 28 and 32°C with high humidity. This reduces the increase in basal metabolic rate due to decreased heat and water loss.

Murphy P. *Essays & MCQs in Anaesthesia and Intensive Care.* Edward Arnold, Chapter 13.
Craft TM, Nolan JP, Parr MJA. *Key Topics in Critical Care.* BIOS Scientific Publishers.

A 60. **A.** true   **B.** true   **C.** true   **D.** false   **E.** false

Hypothermia is defined as a core temperature below 35°C. ECG changes include progressive bradycardia, prolongation of the PR and QT interval, widening of the QRS complex (a late sign) and the appearance of the 'J wave'. Unconsciousness occurs below 30°C, ventricular fibrillation at 28°C, asystole below 20°C and no cerebral activity below 20°C. On rewarming, defibrillation is unlikely to be successful until the patient has been warmed to a core temperature of 30°C and drugs should be withheld or dose-adjusted until this point because of the risk of accumulation with decreased metabolism at low body temperatures.

Craft TM, Nolan JP, Parr MJA. *Key Topics in Critical Care.* BIOS Scientific Publishers.

A 1.   **A.** false   **B.** true   **C.** false   **D.** true   **E.** true

Severe hypercalcaemia is usually treated medically until plasma calcium is below 3 mmol/L, though emergency parathyroid surgery for life-threatening hypercalcaemia has been reported. Hypercalcaemia leads to a short Q-T interval on the ECG. Medullary carcinoma of the thyroid, hyperparathyroidism and phaeochromocytoma co-exist in patients with the multiple endocrine neoplasia syndrome (type II).

Prys-Roberts, Brown. *International Practice of Anaesthesia*. Butterworth Heinemann, Chapter 82.

A 2.   **A.** true   **B.** false   **C.** true   **D.** false   **E.** false

More hypotension occurs when adrenaline-containing local anaesthetics are used for epidural blockade. This may be due to the β_2-effects of the absorbed adrenaline causing vasodilation in peripheral beds. It is countered by the chronotropic and inotropic effects on β_1-receptors. However, the more prolonged hypotension seen is probably due to the achievement of a more profound degree of sympathetic blockade. Sympathetic blockade occurs after sensory blockade. Small unmyelinated sensory fibres with no barrier to local anaesthetic diffusion are blocked before the larger autonomic B fibres. Anterior spinal artery syndrome is due to severe hypotension secondary to epidural blockade and not due to the technique itself. This leads to infarction of the spinal cord and results in a lower motor neurone paralysis at the level of the lesion and spastic paraplegia with decreased pain and temperature sensation below the level. Epidural blockade may cause lower intercostal muscle and abdominal muscle weakness resulting in impaired coughing and exhalation. However, with a T4 block diaphragmatic innervation (C3–C5) is maintained and tidal volume and inspiratory pressure are maintained. Bowel contraction results from blockade of the sympathetic outflow and unopposed parasympathetic activity. Sphincters relax and peristalsis increases.

Barash, Cullen, Stoelting. Clinical Anaesthesia. Chapter 30.

A 3. **A.** false **B.** true **C.** false **D.** false **E.** false

The tare weight is the weight of an empty cylinder plus valve block. It is stamped on the side of the valve block and is used for calculation of the contents of the cylinder by weight. N_2O, cyclopropane and CO_2 cylinders contain liquid. N_2O cylinders are pressurised to 40 bar maximum at 15°C (O_2 cylinders are 137 bar). A size E oxygen cylinder contains 680 L, whereas a size E N_2O cylinder contains 1,800 L.

Yentis, Hirsch, Smith. Anaesthesia A to Z. Butterworth Heinemann, 1993.

A 4. **A.** true **B.** true **C.** false **D.** true **E.** false

These are common drugs that you probably use almost every day. You should know how they are presented. Of the relaxants, suxamethonium and mivacurium are the only chlorides. All the...curoniums are bromides, and...atracuriums are besylates. Gallamine triethiodide is the odd one out. Although fentanyl is a citrate, alfentanil and remifentanil are presented as hydrochlorides. Neostigmine is a methylsulphate, atropine is a sulphate, glycopyrronium is a bromide. All the amide local anaesthetics are hydrochlorides, as is ketamine and most of the inotropes. However, noradrenaline and adrenaline are acid tartrates.

British National Formulary.

A 5. **A.** false **B.** true **C.** false **D.** true **E.** false

A circle system has SEVEN components: 1) Fresh gas inflow, 2) inspiratory and expiratory valves, 3) breathing tubing, 4) Y-connector, 5) APL valve, 6) reservoir bag and 7) absorbent. To prevent rebreathing of CO_2 THREE basic rules need to be observed: 1) Unidirectional valves need to be located on both limbs between the patient and the reservoir bag, 2) FGF must not enter between the expiratory valve and the patient, 3) APL must not be sited between the patient and the inspiratory valve. The system can be semi-open, semi-closed, or closed depending on FGF. Semi-open has no rebreathing but requires a very high fresh gas flow. Most are used as semi-closed systems when a degree of rebreathing is allowed following CO_2 absorption. In a closed system FGF matches uptake of O_2 and agent by the patient. The circle system has many arrangements but the most efficient, which allows the highest conservation of fresh gas is one with the one-way valves near the patient and the adjustable pressure-limiting valve just downstream from the expiratory valve. Sticking of these valves can be a problem. Rebreathing occurs if the valves stick in the open position, whereas total occlusion of the circuit can occur if the valves are stuck closed. Sevoflurane degrades in baralyme and soda lime at a rate directly related to temperature. It does not, however, appear to produce any toxic effects. Phenolphthalein is an indicator that can be used to indicate absorbent exhaustion; it changes from white to pink.

Barash, Cullen, Stoelting. *Clinical Anaesthesia*, 2nd Edn. Chapter 25.
Miller RD. *Anaesthesia*, 5th Edn. Churchill Livingstone.

A 6. **A.** true **B.** false **C.** false **D.** true **E.** true

Previous myocardial infarction, congestive cardiac failure, hypertension, peripheral vascular disease and the presence of preoperative dysrhythmias (non-sinus rhythm or more than five premature ventricular contractions/min) have all been identified as independent risk factors for perioperative cardiac morbidity. Despite the association of diabetes mellitus with atherosclerosis and ischaemic heart disease, most studies have not found it to be an independent risk factor for cardiac morbidity. Regardless of the presence of angiographically significant coronary artery disease, several studies have failed to identify stable angina as an independent risk factor or have found it to be a risk factor only when co-existing with congestive cardiac failure.

Goldhill, Strunin. *Clinical Anaesthesiology: The High Risk Surgical Patient*. Bailliere, Chapter 1.

A 7. **A.** false **B.** false **C.** false **D.** false **E.** false

In general, drugs for hypertension, angina or arrhythmias should be continued throughout the perioperative period in patients scheduled to undergo non-cardiac surgery. There is evidence to suggest that this practice helps prevent perioperative cardiovascular complications and avoids the acute withdrawal syndromes that have occasionally been reported. The antiarrhythmic agent amiodarone has been associated with reports of perioperative bradycardia, profound vasodilatation, low cardiac output and death. However, preoperative discontinuation is not recommended given the risk of recurrence of the underlying dysrhythmia and because, given its long half-life (approx. 35 days), it would need to be stopped some months before surgery. Long-term low-dose aspirin therapy is the mainstay of secondary prevention in patients with underlying atherosclerotic disease. On the basis of current limited evidence that there is an increased incidence of significant perioperative bleeding, it is generally advised that patients undergoing a TURP should have their aspirin therapy discontinued preoperatively. To permit a sufficient recovery of platelet function, this needs to be done at least 7–10 days before surgery. A recent study has suggested that patients, with or at risk of coronary heart disease, who are scheduled to undergo non-cardiac surgery, may benefit from perioperative therapy with the β-blocker atenolol. Thiazide and loop diuretics need not be omitted on the day of surgery although they can cause hypokalaemia, which should be identified and corrected before surgery. Hypertensive patients receiving enalapril, an angiotensin converting enzyme (ACE) inhibitor, may have a higher risk of hypotension on induction of anaesthesia. To date there is no evidence to suggest that this has an adverse effect on long-term outcome and it is therefore probably acceptable for ACE inhibitors to be continued with care perioperatively.

Drugs in the perioperative period. *Drug and Therapeutics Bulletin (1999).* Volume 37. Number 12.

A 8. **A.** false **B.** false **C.** false **D.** false **E.** false

During one-lung anaesthesia although the lower (dependent) lung receives the major portion of pulmonary blood flow and the entire minute ventilation, the upper, unventilated lung will continue to receive a varying proportion of right ventricular cardiac output. Calculated intrapulmonary shunt (true anatomical shunt combined with the physiologic shunt due to ventilation-perfusion mismatching) therefore varies between 30 and 40% when the upper lung is collapsed. This increase in intrapulmonary shunt (venous admixture) will in turn result in impaired carbon dioxide excretion. However, the effect is counterbalanced by a reduction in the dead space:tidal volume ratio. Therefore, providing minute ventilation remains constant, carbon dioxide elimination will remain essentially unchanged on switching to one-lung ventilation. Paradoxically, hypoxaemia is particularly common if the collapsed upper lung is normal or the dependent lower lung abnormal. (A diseased lung, even if it has a focal lesion, tends to have a reduced blood supply.) Hypoxaemia will be further worsened if compensatory hypoxic pulmonary vasoconstriction (HPV) is insufficient to maintain adequate oxygen exchange. While *in vitro* experiments have clearly demonstrated that inhalational anaesthetic agents inhibit HPV this has not been conclusively shown to be the case *in vivo*. This is thought to be because they reduce cardiac output and, in so doing, indirectly enhance the HPV response. There, therefore, appears to be an unchanged HPV response in the presence of volatile anaesthetic agents during one-lung anaesthesia. true anatomical shunt describes that portion of the cardiac output that passes from the right ventricle to the systemic circulation without coming into contact with alveolar gas. This amounts to approximately 5% in normal subjects but increases markedly in pathological conditions where there is lung collapse. In contrast to physiologic shunt, hypoxaemia due to true anatomical shunt is little affected by an increase in the FiO_2 alone. In this situation, application of PEEP to the dependent lung and continuous positive airway pressure (CPAP) to the collapsed upper lung while ensuring large tidal volumes (airway pressures permitting) may prove more beneficial in limiting the subsequent hypoxaemia that results when lung units collapse.

Gothard, Kelleher. *Essentials of Cardiac and Thoracic Anaesthesia.* Butterworth Heinemann, Chapter 7.

A 9.   **A.** true   **B.** true   **C.** true   **D.** false   **E.** true

There is a high proportion of children presenting for GA day case dental work. They are unpremedicated and anxious. Arrhythmias are common especially with the use of halothane and made worse with the use of 1 in 80,000 adrenaline infiltration solutions. Their incidence is reduced with intermittent positive pressure ventilation. The Jorgensen technique using pentobarbitone, pethidine and hyoscine is a recognised sedation technique which maintains cardiovascular stability but may delay recovery. The Goldman nasal mask is a black, inflatable, rimmed mask which is often used. It allows access to the mouth. It has an adjustable pressure-limiting valve and attaches to the breathing system over the patient's forehead. The McKesson's mask is another nasal mask. Maxillary and mandibular nerve blocks may be used to perform dental surgery. Cardiovascular collapse has occurred following these blocks. Suggested causes include retrograde flow of local anaesthetic via branches of the external carotid artery reaching the internal carotid artery, or perineural spread to the medulla. The sitting position is most familiar to dentists, but there is a fear of fainting during anaesthesia and cardiovascular collapse. The reclining position, with the foot of the chair raised, is a compromise between the sitting and supine position.

Yentis, Hirsch, Smith. *Anaesthesia A to Z*. Butterworth Heinemann.

A 10. A. false   **B.** false   **C.** true   **D.** true   **E.** true

During laser surgery all theatre personnel should wear protective goggles since the eyes are very susceptible to damage. The wavelengths used vary: most in ENT are CO_2 lasers which emit in the infrared wavelengths at 10.6 μm. The most serious potential patient danger is airway fire. An endotracheal tube filled with oxygen at high gas flows acts like a blow-torch in the case of a fire. Non-metal tubes will potentially ignite. N_2O will also support combustion. No one type of ETT will guarantee protection against laser damage. Neodymium-doped yttrium-aluminium-garnet lasers (Nd:YAG) produce energy at 1.06 μm and have greater ability to penetrate tissue than CO_2 lasers. They will easily cut through metal ETTs. If an airway fire occurs, ventilation and oxygen flow should be stopped and the ETT removed immediately. The fire should be extinguished immediately with water or saline and the airway re-secured. Steroids and humidified gases should be used and the patient admitted to ITU for observation.

Barash, Cullen, Stoelting. *Clinical Anesthesia*, 2nd Edn. Chapter 39.

A 11. A. false   **B.** true   **C.** false   **D.** true   **E.** true

Penlon's left-handed laryngoscope is not for left-handed anaesthetists but for use in those patients in whom the nature of dentition or maxilla make it undesirable to exert pressure upon a particular area. Small pieces of equipment may be sterilised by boiling for 5 min. This procedure is suitable for pieces made from metal, rubber or neoprene. Precautions should include boiling for exactly the right time and not reducing the temperature or allowing the possibility of cross-contamination by introducing other pieces of equipment. The oxygen flush bypass is mounted at the end of the backbar. Here it is operated even with a volatile turned on. The patient will receive 100% oxygen, uncontaminated by volatile/nitrous oxide at a rate of 35 l/min. The tracheal tube adaptor is the official term for 'catheter mount'. The latter term does not appear in BS 6015 (ISO 4135), which is the official glossary of terms in anaesthesia. These connectors (also International standard) are 22 mm and have largely replaced older McKesson and MIE 23-mm connectors. They also all taper in the same way with the male taper upstream and female downstream. Passive scavenging systems consist of a tube passing through a wall or roof of the building terminating in an outside vent. They rely upon the wind to entrain and void exhaust gases. Usually the vent is in the roof and as waste gases pass to cooler areas above theatre, they become denser and slower and water vapour may condense to run back down. A water trap is therefore essential.

Ward CS. *Anaesthetic Equipment. Physical Principles and Maintenance.* Balliere Tindall, 2nd Edn.

A 12. A. false **B.** false **C.** true **D.** true **E.** true

Regional anaesthesia has not been shown to reduce the risks of postoperative strokes, although there is some evidence that it may reduce the incidence of perioperative MI. It does however allow for neurological status to be assessed during surgery. If no deterioration occurs after carotid artery occlusion for up to 4 min then shunting is unnecessary and complications (e.g. plaque dislodgement associated with shunting) are avoided. Post operative TIAs are caused most commonly by carotid artery occlusion rather than microemboli. Treatment is heparinisation, increasing blood pressure and re-exploration. Injection of local anaesthetic into the vertebral artery during deep cervical plexus block produces loss of consciousness and seizures. There are many monitors of the adequacy of cerebral perfusion. The stump pressure is a direct measurement of arterial pressure in the ipsilateral carotid artery, measured on the brain-side to a cross clamp placed on the internal carotid artery. It is one of the 'oldest' monitors to be used. One could argue that cerebral perfusion will also be reduced by downstream venous pressure, hence the need to avoid venous occlusion at the site of surgery and contralateral kinking of major veins by excessive turning of the head. The carotid bodies at the bifurcation of the common carotid artery stimulate the respiratory centre in the medulla when CO_2 or hydrogen ion concentration rises and respond to a decrease in O_2. Patients lose their carotid body function and hence lack respiratory stimulation to hypoxia with bilateral, not unilateral, endarterectomy.

Kaplan. *Vascular Anaesthesia*. Churchill Livingstone.

A **13. A.** false **B.** true **C.** false **D.** true **E.** true

The primary drug used preoperatively is an α-blocker. β-blockers are only introduced if necessary. Half-life of plasma catecholamines is approximately 5 min. Prior to the 1950s, refractory hypotension was frequently seen after tumour removal due to the short half-life of secreted catecholamines and chronic hypovolaemia.

Prys-Roberts, Brown. *International Practice of Anaesthesia*. Butterworth Heinemann, Chapter 83.

A **14. A.** true **B.** false **C.** true **D.** true **E.** true

During head-down tilt the endotracheal tube may move down into the right main bronchus, hence its position should be checked after the patient is positioned. Haemodynamic studies have shown a decrease in cardiac output during peritoneal insufflation regardless of head up/down/level position. The cause is multifactorial; an increase in intra-abdominal pressure resulting in blood pooling in the legs and decreasing inferior vena cava blood flow and venous return, an increase in systemic vascular resistance secondary to sympathetic stimulation, increased venous resistance and also a release of catecholamines, prostaglandins and vasopressin. Pneumothorax, pneumoperitoneum and pneumopericardium can all occur during laparoscopy and with intra-abdominal insufflation of gas. Pneumothorax develops through pleural tears during surgery at the gastro-oesophageal junction. There is an increase in $PaCO_2$ with nitrous oxide as the insufflating gas. This is because of the V/Q mismatch and increased physiological dead space secondary to abdominal distension, patient position and reduced cardiac output. Direct intraperitoneal absorption of CO_2 increases $PaCO_2$ when it is used as the insufflating gas. Nerve damage has been reported secondary to patient malposition during laparoscopic procedures. The common peroneal nerve must be protected in the lithotomy position. During prolonged cases, damage to it can lead to lower extremity compartment syndrome. It maybe due to tight leg straps, dorsiflexion of the foot or inadvertent surgical pressure.

Cucchiara, Miller, Reves, Roizen, Savarese. *Anesthesia*, 4th Edn. Churchill Livingstone, Chapter 60.

A 15. **A.** false   **B.** false   **C.** true   **D.** false   **E.** false

The OAA and AAGBI have published guidelines for obstetric anaesthesia services in September 1998. These booklets are available from the AAGBI and should be read prior to the exam. These guidelines include recommendations such as: all obstetric units should have at least 2 units of uncrossmatched O negative blood and that crossmatched blood should be available within 30 min of receiving the blood sample. Although the patient whom the anaesthetist is directly involved with has paramount importance, if it is essential for him/her to leave the patient to deal with a life-threatening emergency nearby (which is a matter of individual judgement), they may do so only if they instruct another person to observe the patient's vital signs and delegate overall responsibility to another registered medical practitioner. There is no difference between the principle of obtaining consent for obstetric anaesthesia and any other medical treatment. Hence consent may be implied or expressed and it may be written or oral. Foetal distress needing anaesthesia for operative delivery requires a short response time. It is recommended that there should not be more than 30 min from informing the anaesthetist to start of operation. All postoperative patients must be continually observed for at least 30 min and until discharge criteria are met. Midwives who

Exam 4

Answers

perform this task must be specifically trained in monitoring, care of the airway and resuscitation procedures.

Guidelines for Obstetric Anaesthetic Services. AAGBI, September 1998.

A 16. **A.** true   **B.** false   **C.** true   **D.** false   **E.** true

Numerous simple, bedside clinical tests have been designed to aid with the diagnosis of a potentially difficult endotracheal intubation. All suffer from relatively poor specificity and sensitivity but it has been suggested that their predictive value may be further enhanced when interpreted in conjunction with a lateral radiograph of the skull and cervical spine in the neutral position. Abnormalities of the shape of the mandible can make direct laryngoscopy difficult. An increased posterior depth of the mandible (measured from the alveolus immediately behind the third molar tooth to the lower border of the mandible) has been shown to hinder displacement of the soft tissues by the blade of the laryngoscope. It has also been determined that an increased anterior depth of the mandible (measured from the tip of the lower incisors to the anterior limit of the lower border of the mandible) may also predispose to a difficult intubation. The degree of extension of the head attainable during intubation is related to the size of the atlanto-occipital gap (measured from the occiput to the spine of the atlas vertebra) in the neutral position. If the gap is reduced, attempts at head extension will result in anterior bowing of the cervical spine and anterior displacement of the larynx. An absent atlanto-axial gap has also been found to be a useful predictor of difficulty when direct laryngoscopy is planned. Thyromental distance (Patil test), describes the distance between the mental prominence (tip of chin) and the thyroid notch with the neck fully extended. A distance <6 cm has been found to be strongly predictive of difficulty with laryngoscopy and/or intubation.

Murphy P. *Essays & MCQs in Anaesthesia and Intensive Care.* Edward Arnold, Chapter 14.

A 17. **A.** true   **B.** true   **C.** false   **D.** true   **E.** false

Fall in measured plasma concentration of an infused drug (and clinical effects) will depend on excretion from the body, distribution to other compartments and redistribution back from these compartments. For infusions of short duration, drugs with the most rapid onset have a small apparent volume of distribution and low rate constant for redistribution. These drugs will have a rapid offset if they are also rapidly excreted. Many drugs also have a rapid offset as a result of extensive redistribution. However, this process leads to a progressive rise in concentration of the drug within body compartments over time unless matched by a high excretion rate. Context-sensitive half-time is a measure of the net effect of these various processes as represented by the time taken for plasma concentration to halve in the context of duration of infusion of the drug. It is less variable for drugs with a low Vdss and low rate constant for redistribution but a high clearance attributable to excretion. Remifentanil satisfies these criteria because of a low Vdss and rapid ester hydrolysis. Fentanyl has an extremely variable context-sensitive half-time. When compared to alfentanil, it has a slower onset because of differences in pKa (8.5 for fentanyl and 6.4 for alfentanil). This means that alfentanil is 100 times less ionised upon injection and reaches the receptor faster. However alfentanil has a much lower Vdss and a slower clearance rate. This means that for short duration infusions (up to 2 h) fentanyl concentration will fall MORE rapidly due to enhanced excretion AND loss from the plasma via redistribution. However, alfentanil reaches its maximum context-sensitive half-time after just 90 min, whereas fentanyl keeps on rising and then overtakes alfentanil due to its massive redistribution potential. Hence nobody uses fentanyl for ITU sedation and analgesia.

Pharmacokinetics of drug infusions. Hill SA. *Continuing Education in Anaesthesia, Critical Care & Pain*. BJA publications, Volume 4, Number 3, June 2004.

A 18. **A.** false **B.** true **C.** true **D.** true **E.** false

Vitamins A, D, E and K are fat soluble. Cholecalciferol (vitamin D3) is 25-hydroxylated in the liver and then converted into the physiologically active 1,25-dihydroxycholecalciferol in the kidney.

Kumar, Clark. *Clinical Medicine*, 3rd Edn. Saunders, Chapter 3.

A 19. **A.** true **B.** false **C.** true **D.** false **E.** false

Ketamine is a phencyclidine derivative. It is only about 12% protein bound, redistribution is slow and metabolism in the liver produces norketamine, an active metabolite. It dilates bronchial muscle and maintains a patent airway. It has been used by infusion to treat severe asthma attacks. Laryngeal and pharyngeal reflexes are maintained but airway secretions may be profuse. It is a central sympathetic stimulant but it depresses the peripheral sympathetic system. Clinically it increases cardiac output and heart rate but arrhythmias are uncommon. Skeletal muscle tone and intraocular pressure are increased.

Smith, Aitkenhead. *Textbook of anaesthesia*. Churchill Livingstone.

A 20. A. true **B.** true **C.** true **D.** false **E.** true

Thiopentone is 80% protein bound. Its elimination follows first-order kinetics, which may become zero order at higher doses. It can and has been given rectally as a 5 or 10% solution. It may cause a tachycardia due to a decrease in vagal tone. Perivascular injection may cause tissue necrosis and damage is limited with hyaluronidase. Recommended treatments for intra-arterial injection include papaverine, stellate ganglion or brachial plexus block as well as heparin and oral anticoagulants.

Smith, Aitkenhead. *Textbook of anaesthesia*. Churchill Livingstone.

A 21. A. false **B.** false **C.** true **D.** true **E.** true

Hypocapnia ($PaCO_2$ <4.7 kPa) is caused by hyperventilation. It leads to alkalosis, hence hypokalaemia, hypocalcaemia and tetany; vasoconstriction, hence reduced placental and cerebral blood flow. These in turn cause dizziness and confusion in the conscious, or convulsions in the pre-disposed.

Yentis, Hirsch, Smith. *Anaesthesia A to Z*. Butterworth Heinemann, 1993.

A 22. A. true **B.** false **C.** true **D.** false **E.** true

The hepatic artery is a branch of the coeliac axis. There is an inverse ratio of the flow between the hepatic artery and portal vein, but under normal conditions 1/3 of hepatic blood comes from the hepatic artery. β_2-adrenergic receptors mediate vasodilation. Portal blood flow does not autoregulate well. PEEP increases hepatic venous pressure and reduces portal flow.

The countercurrent exchange of oxygen between parallel arterioles and submucosal venules makes oxygen delivery to the tips of mucosal villi poor. The splanchnic and skin circulations are the major reservoirs of available blood in times of stress.

Reitan J, Kien N in *Cardiovascular Physiology*. Priebe HJ and Skarvan K (eds). BMJ Publishing Group, 1995.

A 23. A. true **B.** false **C.** true **D.** false **E.** true

Absorption of bile salts occurs in the terminal ileum, and of iron in the duodenum and jejunum.

Kumar, Clark. *Clinical Medicine*, 3rd Edn. Saunders, Chapter 5.

A 24. A. true **B.** true **C.** false **D.** true **E.** false

The lungs store approximately 3,000 ml (FRC = RV + ERV) after breathing 100% oxygen. Oxygen delivery (DO_2) equals cardiac output multiplied by arterial oxygen content (CaO_2). Uptake may be estimated by multiplying cardiac output by arterio-venous oxygen content difference.

Prys-Roberts, Brown. *International Practice of Anaesthesia*. Butterworth Heinemann, Chapter 61.

A 25. A. true **B.** true **C.** false **D.** false **E.** true

Mu opioid receptors inhibit adenylyl cyclase. Histamine receptors are found throughout the CNS (antihistamines have both sedating and antinauseant properties due to their effects on the CNS).

Prys-Roberts, Brown. *International Practice of Anaesthesia*. Butterworth Heinemann, Chapter 7.

A 26. A. true **B.** true **C.** true **D.** false **E.** true

Codeine requires metabolism by a cytochrome enzyme system to be activated to morphine. This is unfortunately not possible for some individuals due to genetic variability in these enzymes. Combined preparations, for example, with 8 mg of codeine, as are commonly available, do not significantly reduce pain compared to paracetamol alone but do induce constipation. Use of paracetamol as an adjunct to codeine treatment alone does significantly improve efficacy. Number needed to treat to achieve a 50% reduction in pain score using codeine 60 mg alone = 16.7; a combined preparation of codeine 60 mg + paracetamol 1 g = 2.2. Compare these NNT values with other agents: morphine 10 mg = 2.9, ibuprofen 400 mg = 2.4, ketorolac 30 mg = 3.4 and diclofenac 50 mg = 2.0.

Rawal N. *Management of Acute and Chronic Pain.* BMJ Books, 1998.

A 27. A. false **B.** true **C.** false **D.** true **E.** true

Kerley 'B' lines are oedematous interlobular septa. Without chronic pulmonary vessel changes, vessel redistribution occurs between 16 and 22 cmH$_2$O, interstitial oedema between 22 and 30 cmH$_2$O and alveolar oedema after 30 cmH$_2$O. The main pulmonary artery forms the border between the aortic knuckle and the left atrial appendage. In more than 70% of patients a cardiothoracic ratio of >55% is associated with an ejection fraction of <40%.

Wilson A. *Medicine* 1997;25:10–18.
Hull J, Bion F in *Handbook of Clinical Anaesthesia.* Goldstone J, Pollard B (eds). Churchill Livingstone, 1996.

A 28. A. false **B.** false **C.** true **D.** true **E.** true

The EEG only records the electrical activity of the pyramidal cells in the superficial cortical laminae. Carbamazapine is an enzyme inducer and its interactions should be remembered. Phenytoin is an antiarrhythmic as well as anticonvulsant drug. It causes hypotension after rapid infusion because of its diluents, usually propylene glycol and ethanol, and because of direct cardiac depression. The effects of anaesthetics on epilepsy and EEG and varying concentrations are complicated. It is generally accepted that enflurane particularly at >1.5 MAC with hypocarbia may help localise epileptic foci for surgical intervention. Butyrophenones and phenothiazines lower the threshold for seizures. This warning usually appears when they are used as antipsychotic drugs rather than antiemetics.

A. true   **B.** true   **C.** false   **D.** false   **E.** false

Hepatitis A has an incubation period of 2–3 weeks. It does not lead to chronic liver disease or a carrier state, and has an acute mortality of <0.5%.

Kumar, Clark. *Clinical Medicine*, 3rd Edn. Saunders, Chapter 5.

A 30. **A.** true   **B.** false   **C.** true   **D.** true   **E.** true

Dystrophia myotonica is a systemic disease characterised by an inability to relax after voluntary muscle contraction OR in response to mechanical stimulation of the muscle. There is muscle weakness and atrophy. Associated findings include cataracts, frontal balding, gonadal atrophy, cholelithiasis and intellectual changes. Typical features include facial weakness, pharyngeal dystrophy, delayed gastric emptying because of poor smooth muscle motility and cardiomyopathy with conduction disorders. There may be respiratory muscle weakness and death from cardiorespiratory failure. The cause is an underlying abnormality of calcium metabolism allowing continued contractility. Suxamethonium may result in severe myotonia and should be avoided. Neostigmine, halothane and shivering may also produce myotonia. Regional procedures do not reduce the risk of myotonia.

Nimmo, Rowbotham, Smith. *Anaesthesia*, 2nd Edn. Volume 2.

A 31. **A.** true   **B.** false   **C.** false   **D.** false   **E.** true

Sarcoidosis typically causes bilateral hilar lymphadenopathy. The Kveim test (intradermal injection of sarcoid tissue) is no longer used because of the risk of infection.

A 32. **A.** true   **B.** false   **C.** true   **D.** true   **E.** false

Myasthenia gravis affects proximal limbs more than distal and upper more than lower. Respiratory weakness is unusual unless myasthenic or cholinergic crises intervene. In the younger age groups (10–40 years), females are more commonly affected, whereas there is an equal sex distribution in the older age groups. Receptor lifespan is shortened. About 15% have a thymoma and thymectomy results in remission in 60–80% but occasionally after a delay of several years. Diagnosis is made by a reduction in single twitch height and a decreased response to tetanic or repeated stimuli on EMG. Muscle weakness may be precipitated by aminoglycosides, infection, electrolyte abnormalities, pregnancy and surgical stress. Treatment is with anticholinesterases, pyridostigmine being longer acting with fewer muscarinic side effects than neostigmine. Both cholinergic excess and deficiency may occur at the same time in different muscle groups. Volatile agents affect the neuromuscular junction and may reduce twitch height unlike those without the condition. Isoflurane may be better than halothane because it is excreted more rapidly. Suxamethonium may result in a non-depolarising block. All non-depolarisers cause an increased degree of block and some produce a block of longer duration. Anticholinesterase therapy should be continued up until the time of operation and recommenced as soon as possible afterwards.

Nimmo, Rowbotham, Smith. *Anaesthesia*, 2nd Edn. Volume 2.

A 33. A. false   **B.** false   **C.** true   **D.** false   **E.** false

Haemophilia A is an X-linked disease. The bleeding time is normal and predominantly tests platelet function. The activated partial thromboplastin time is prolonged. 50% of haemophilia carriers have levels of factor VIII sufficient to warrant haematological prophylaxis prior to major surgery. DDAVP (Deamino-D-arginine vasopressin) can raise factor VIII levels in mild haemophiliacs to cover minor surgery. DDAVP takes 1 h to act and increases endogenous Factor VIII and von Willibrand Factor as well as tissue plasminogen activator so it is sometimes administered with an antifibrinolytic such as tranexamic acid. Factor VIII usually has a half-life of 8 h. Synthetic Factor VIII may have a shorter half-life or be ineffective because of antibodies in haemophiliacs.

Hoffbrand A. *Postgraduate Haematology*, 4th Edn. Butterworth Heinemann, 1998.

A 34. A. true   **B.** true   **C.** true   **D.** true   **E.** false

The left common iliac vein is crossed by the right common iliac artery and ovarian arteries which together with presence of the gravid uterus may predispose to left-sided thrombosis. Elevated factor VIII levels in pregnancy may explain why APTT is an unreliable monitor for appropriate heparin dosing in pregnancy. The radiation dose to the foetus from a ventilation-perfusion scan is deemed to pose a negligible risk.

Greer I. *Lancet* 1999;353:1258–1265.

A 35. **A.** false **B.** true **C.** true **D.** true **E.** true

A Le Fort I fracture just involves the palate and maxillary antra. The mortality for children requiring re-operation for bleeding following tonsillectomy and adenoidectomy is approximately 1 in 500. Recent meta-analyses (2004) suggest that re-bleeding rates have been increased by the use of disposable/single-use instruments such as diathermy. These instruments were introduced following DoH advice to minimise the theoretical risk of vCJD transmission during operations on lymphoid tissue, but have probably increased overall risk associated with tonsillectomy in the UK.

Prys-Roberts, Brown. *International Practice of Anaesthesia*, 1st Edn. Butterworth Heinemann, Chapters 109 and 112.

A 36. **A.** false **B.** false **C.** true **D.** true **E.** true

A Hartmann's procedure results in a proximal colostomy with oversewing of the distal bowel. Low rectal carcinomas are treated with an abdomino-perineal resection.

A 37. **A.** true **B.** false **C.** true **D.** false **E.** true

Therapeutic magnesium levels are 4–6 mg/dL not per litre. Always check the units quoted as well as the figures, this is an easy mistake to make! Foetuses with occiput posterior can still have a spontaneous delivery, though instrumental delivery is often necessary. The death rate associated with Caesarean section (from all causes) in the UK and USA is approximately 1 in 2,000.

Prys-Roberts, Brown. *International Practice of Anaesthesia*. Butterworth Heinemann, Chapters 97 and 98.

A 38. A. false **B.** true **C.** false **D.** false **E.** true

The skin over the thyroid is supplied by the cervical plexus. Deep block of this plexus may affect the phrenic nerve and paralyse the diaphragm. Hypocalcaemia should be quickly ruled out as a cause of laryngospasm occurring between 24 and 48 h after surgery. Most retrosternal goitres can still be excised via a standard incision. Multiple endocrine neoplasia type 2 predisposes to parathyroid tumours, medullary carcinoma of the thyroid and phaeochromocytoma.

Anaesthesia and the endocrine system. Barash P, Cullen B, Stoelting R. *Clinical Anaesthesia*, 3rd Edn. Lippincott-Raven, 1997.

A 39. A. true **B.** true **C.** false **D.** false **E.** false

Necrotising enterocolitis (NEC) has a mortality of 55%. Its incidence varies from 1.1 to 2.4 per 1,000 live births. It classically occurs in the premature and low birth weight child but may occur in full-term infants. It is caused by intestinal mucosal injury from reduced mesenteric blood flow. Unless there is evidence of necrosis (gangrene from a positive paracentesis) or perforation (pneumoperitoneum), the initial treatment is conservative. Relative indications for surgery include clinical deterioration (acidosis, respiratory failure, oliguria, leucopaenia), portal vein gas, erythema of the abdominal wall, a fixed abdominal mass or a persistently dilated loop of bowel.

Motoyama, Davis, Mosby. *Smith's Anesthesia for Infants and Children*, 6th Edn. Chapter 14.

A 40. A. false **B.** true **C.** true **D.** true **E.** false

Decreased secretion: insulin, testosterone, oestrogen and T3.
Unchanged secretion: TSH, LH and FSH.
Increased secretion: GH, ACTH, β-endorphin, prolactin, ADH, catecholamines, cortisol, aldosterone, glucagon and renin.
The stress response comes up time and again in both MCQs and Viva examinations. It is difficult to modify the response clinically. Opioids suppress hypothalamic and pituitary hormone secretion, but it takes doses of >50 μg/kg fentanyl to abolish response to pelvic and abdominal surgery. Etomidate suppresses adrenal corticosteroid production by reversible inhibition of

11-β-hydroxylase. An induction dose of 0.3 mg/kg blocks aldosterone and cortisol production for up to 8 h. Central neural blockade can reduce the glucose, ACTH, cortisol, GH and adrenaline changes associated with surgery.

Endocrine and metabolic response to surgery. Burton D, Nicholson G, Hall G. Continuing Education in Anaesthesia, Critical Care & Pain. BJA publications, Volume 4, Number 5, October 2004.

A 41. A. false   **B.** false   **C.** false   **D.** true   **E.** true

The ECG is useful as a heart rate monitor in arrhythmia detection and to identify ischaemia. It does not provide a continuous monitor of circulation, as demonstrated by a pulseless electrical activity (PEA) arrest (EMD). Standard lead II monitors the right coronary artery region, best for ischaemia. It is used for providing the best P wave, and is therefore the best rhythm monitor. Trans-oesophageal echocardiography has demonstrated that the majority of ischaemic incidents go undetected on the ECG. CM5 monitoring is a modified lead V5 view that monitors the left ventricle for ischaemia. Lead positions are as above, with the right arm electrode placed over the manubrium sternum and the ground electrode placed on the left shoulder. Chest leads V4-V6 monitor the circumflex artery territory.

Nimmo, Rowbotham, Smith. *Anaesthesia*, 2nd Edn. Blackwell Scientific Publications, Chapter 35.

A 42. A. true   **B.** false   **C.** false   **D.** true   **E.** true

The Wright's respirometer is an anemometer, i.e. it measures gas velocity. It is a simple mechanical device and tends to under-read at low flows and over-read at high flows due to the inertia/momentum of the vane, respectively. It can be placed in the 'to-and-fro' part of a breathing system as it only measures gas flow in one direction. The Datex Ultima monitor uses two Pitot tubes to measure velocity of gas flow in both directions within a circuit. A pitot tube is a cylindrical open-ended tube that measures stagnation pressure. One is faced upstream and the other downstream. The monitor also samples gas composition to correct for density and viscosity. Other flowmeters are available, including thermistor systems, where the cooling effect of gas flow on a thermistor is measured, and ultrasonic systems where the frequency of the oscillation of turbulent eddies formed around a rod in the gas path is measured using a Doppler probe.

Yentis, Hirsch, Smith. *Anaesthesia A to Z*. Butterworth Heinemann.
Miller RD. *Anesthesia*, 5th Edn. Churchill Livingstone.

A **43.** **A.** true **B.** false **C.** true **D.** false **E.** false

Boyle's law states that, at a constant temperature, the volume of a given mass of gas varies inversely with its absolute pressure. Charles's law states that, at constant pressure, the volume of a given mass of gas varies directly with the absolute temperature. The third gas law states that at constant volume the absolute pressure of a given mass of gas varies directly with absolute temperature. Dalton's law of partial pressures states that in a mixture of gases the pressure exerted by each gas is the same as that which it would exert if it alone occupied the container. 101.3 kPa is equal to 760 mmHg. Avogadro's hypothesis states that equal volumes of gases at the same temperature and pressure contain equal numbers of molecules. Adiabatic changes are those that involve changes in the state of a gas without transfer of heat with the surroundings.

Parbrook GD, Davis PD, Parbrook EO. *Basic Physics and Measurement in Anaesthesia*. Heinnemann.

A **44.** **A.** false **B.** true **C.** true **D.** false **E.** false

MAC or minimum alveolar concentration is an unfortunate term. It is conceptually easier to understand if it is regarded as minimum alveolar PARTIAL PRESSURE (MAPP). These values conveniently coincide when concentrations are compared with partial pressures (kPa) at sea level. Variations in inspired concentration or ambient pressure both give rise to changes in alveolar partial pressure of the inhaled agent, but the standard 'MAPP' quoted at sea level will remain valid within the range of ambient pressures used clinically (up to 6 atmospheres). However, even if the required inspired partial pressure remains constant at altitude, the apparent MAC (N.B. CONCENTRATION) of an agent will appear to have risen because the fall in overall ambient pressure will have necessitated an increase in the fractional concentration of the agent to maintain the required partial pressure (Dalton's law of partial pressures). James and White tested Fluotec Mark II and Dräger Vapor halothane vaporisers at sea level, at 5,000 ft and 10,000 ft altitude. At any given setting the delivered percentage of halothane increased with altitude; however, its partial pressure remained constant. Therefore, when these devices are used at a given vaporiser setting, anaesthetic will be delivered at a constant potency regardless of altitude. The TEC 6 vaporiser is specifically designed to deliver desflurane. To overcome the difficulty of unpredictable vaporisation at 20°C (desflurane has a boiling point of 23.5°C), the vaporiser is electrically heated to maintain a constant 39°C in the vaporisation sump. Here, ambient pressure is maintained at 2 atmospheres. Downstream, pressure is autoregulated to maintain a pressure of 1.1 atmospheres at a fresh gas flow of 10 L/min. Therefore, unlike contemporary variable-bypass vaporisers, the Tec 6 vaporiser requires manual adjustments of the concentration control dial at altitudes other than sea level to maintain a constant partial pressure of anaesthetic. Since it is working at its own pressure, altitude does not affect its output, and it will accurately deliver the dialled volumes percent of desflurane, but this does not equal an accurate partial pressure of anaesthetic. To compensate for the reduction in partial pressure, the set concentration on the dial must be increased to maintain the required anaesthetic partial pressure. For example, at an altitude of 2,000 m, the anaesthetist would have to manually increase the concentration control dial from 10 to 12.8% to maintain the required anaesthetic partial pressure.

Miller. *Anaesthesia*, 4th Edn. Chapters 9 and 71.

A 45. A. true **B.** true **C.** false **D.** true **E.** false

A head lift should be sustainable for 5 s. A post-tetanic count of 8 indicates 'surgical' relaxation. Maximum inspiratory pressure of $-35\,cmH_2O$ is considered the minimum acceptable indicator of adequacy of reversal. Some would argue that $-50\,cmH_2O$ is associated with full return of upper airway control. Presence of handgrip, although useful, is also dependent upon the cooperation of an awake patient. Arterial PCO_2 may be raised if the patient is inadequately reversed but in view of all the other possible causes is an insensitive indicator of poor reversal.

Miller. *Anaesthesia*, 4th Edn.

Exam 4

Answers

A 46. A. false **B.** false **C.** false **D.** false **E.** true

The fuel cell consists of a gold mesh cathode and lead anode. The electrolyte is usually potassium hydroxide. Current flow depends on oxygen uptake at the cathode. The cell produces a voltage and does not rely on a battery. The life depends on period of exposure to oxygen, which may be several months. Water vapour has little effect and the cell has a finite but guaranteed lifespan.

Parbrook GD, Davis PD, Parbrook EO. *Basic Physics and Measurement in Anaesthesia*. Heinnemann.

A 47. A. false **B.** true **C.** false **D.** false **E.** false

Digoxin, calcium salts and thyroxine have cAMP-independent positive inotropic effects. As a phosphodiesterase inhibitor, aminophylline does have positive inotropic effects but in practice the clinical dose required is so high as to make the side effects intolerable.

Oh T. *Intensive Care Manual*, 4th Edn. Butterworth Heinemann, Chapter 12.

A 48. A. false **B.** true **C.** false **D.** true **E.** false

Partial pressure to inspired oxygen ratio (PaO_2/FiO_2) $<20\,kPa$, despite a normal $PaCO_2$ and regardless of positive end-expiratory pressure (PEEP) is an accepted diagnostic criterion for ARDS. Pulmonary infiltrates on chest X-ray are bilateral in ARDS and although pulmonary infection may be a precipitating cause its presence is not obligatory to the diagnosis. A PCWP $>18\,mmHg$ suggests that the pulmonary oedema present is cardiac in origin, not an interstitial oedema.

Oh T. *Intensive Care Manual*, 4th Edn. Butterworth Heinemann, Chapter 29.

A 49. A. false **B.** false **C.** true **D.** true **E.** false

The cause of the coma must be established and be considered irreversible. To be diagnosed brain dead, all sedative agents and muscle relaxants must have been discontinued and time allowed for their metabolism and elimination. Hypothermia must be corrected to a core temperature of 35°C in advance of testing the patient. Doll's eye movements will be absent but plantar reflexes and tendon stretch reflexes are of spinal cord origin and so may persist in the presence of brainstem death. Current UK legislation states that once diagnosed brain dead, a patient may then proceed to organ donation if clinically appropriate and the patient has not stated otherwise. Consent is sought from relatives as an act of courtesy, not as a legal requirement.

Oh T. *Intensive Care Manual*, 4th Edn. Butterworth Heinemann, Chapter 45.

A **50.** **A.** true   **B.** true   **C.** false   **D.** false   **E.** false

Anti-HIV antibodies are usually detected in the patient's serum by 12 weeks following infection. However, for patients without detectable anti-HIV antibodies, sera may be positive for p24 antigen (a component of the HIV core protein) or HIV RNA. PCP may occur with any immunodeficiency state and is characterised by fever, dry cough and pleuritic retrosternal chest pain. Meningitis is the most common manifestation of infection with *cryptococcus neoformans* and it is infection with *cryptosporidium*, which affects the gastro-intestinal tract causing severe and intractable secretory diarrhoea.

Oh T. *Intensive Care Manual*, 4th Edn. Butterworth Heinemann, Chapters 59 and 60.

A **51.** **A.** false   **B.** true   **C.** true   **D.** false   **E.** true

Bartter's syndrome (a renal condition affecting the loss of hydrogen ions from the distal tubules) and corticosteroid therapy result in a metabolic alkalosis rather than an acidosis.

Oh T. *Intensive Care Manual*, 4th Edn. Butterworth Heinemann, Chapter 80.

A **52.** **A.** true   **B.** false   **C.** false   **D.** true   **E.** false

Mortality from burns has significantly improved in the last 50 years. It is related to various factors such as surface area and depth of burn, age, co-morbidities and other injuries, particularly inhalational injury. Carbon monoxide has an affinity for haemoglobin 240 times that of oxygen, which together with shifting the oxyhaemoglobin dissociation curve to the left, means there is a considerable reduction in the amount of oxygen available for metabolism. The clinical effects of carbon monoxide

Exam 4

Answers

poisoning depend on the proportion of carboxyhaemoglobin present: tinnitus and headache occur at 10–20%, drowsiness at 20–40% and convulsions, coma and cardiac arrest above 40%. Suxamethonium can be used safely for the initial 24 h after injury.

Oh T. *Intensive Care Manual*, 4th Edn. Butterworth, 1997, Chapter 72. Craft TM, Nolan JP, Parr MJA. *Key Topics in Intensive Care*, 1st Edn. BIOS Scientific Publishers, 1999.

A 53. A. false **B.** true **C.** true **D.** true **E.** false

Guillain Barre syndrome (GBS) is an acute inflammatory demyelinating polyradiculoneuropathy. The diagnosis requires a progressive motor weakness of more than one limb and areflexia or marked hyporeflexia. CSF opening pressure and white cell count are normal but protein levels are typically elevated. Two clinical variants have been described, the axonal form (associated with *C. jejuni*) and the Miller Fisher syndrome (strictly a separate condition but sharing some overlap features with GBS). The former has a worse prognosis.

Oh T. *Intensive Care Manual*, 4th Edn. Butterworth, 1997. Craft TM, Nolan JP, Parr MJA. *Key Topics in Critical Care*, 1st Edn. BIOS Scientific Publishers,1999.

A 54. A. true **B.** true **C.** true **D.** true **E.** true

All these conditions and drugs are known to be associated with acute pancreatitis.

Oh T. *Intensive Care Manual*. 4th Edn. Butterworth Heinemann, Chapter 36.

A 55. A. true **B.** true **C.** false **D.** false **E.** true

In patients with ARF, endogenous urea can be converted to non-essential amino acids if an adequate amount of carbohydrate is provided. The Giordano Giovanetti diet contains a high carbohydrate load with limited protein. The use of commercially available essential amino acids with hypertonic glucose aids control of electrolyte balance, lowers blood urea nitrogen levels, decreases the need for dialysis and speeds recovery of patients with acute tubular necrosis. Using high concentrations of glucose in a small volume allows even an oliguric patient to receive enough calories. Feinstein employed an interesting approach to providing amino acids to patients with haemodialysis-dependent renal failure by including them in the dialysate.

Miller RD. *Anaesthesia*, 4th edn. Chapter 78.

A 56. A. false **B.** true **C.** true **D.** true **E.** false

The first letter of the pacemaker code relates to the chamber paced (Atrium, Ventricle, Dual), the second to the chamber sensed and the third to the response. Remember **PaSemakeR**! For example VVI means that the ventricle is both sensed and paced, and if sensing occurs the pacemaker is inhibited. Unipolar pacemakers have the cathode at the tip, and the anode is the case. Bipolar pacemakers have the anode approximately 2.5 cm from the tip. The threshold is the pacemaker output needed for successful pacing. It is found by gradually decreasing the output until the myocardium fails to contract (failure to capture). Threshold is normally about 0.5–2 V, and the pacemaker wire should be re-sited if it increases above 5 V. Threshold may increase up to threefold in the weeks following insertion.

Kumar, Clark. *Clinical Medicine*, 3rd Edn. Saunders, Chapter 11.

A 57. A. false **B.** true **C.** true **D.** true **E.** false

Hyperventilation with a low $PaCO_2$ is classical at the beginning of an asthma attack. A normal CO_2 indicates reduced alveolar ventilation secondary to an increasing number of lung units with slow time constants. The description of 'volume', 'flow' and 'pressure' dependent collapse of airways is confusing. Pure asthmatics have narrowed airways and a high airway resistance due to increased bronchomotor tone and mucosal oedema. The subsequent fall in airway pressure during flow across the resistance favours collapse. It is a peculiarity of asthma that more capillary blood can come into contact with inspired gas by virtue of altered ventilation perfusion matching and airway inflammation. The actual arterial PO_2 is more likely to decrease. Although a low inspiratory flow rate resulting in a low peak inspiratory pressure is desirable during ventilation, it has been demonstrated that for a given respiratory rate, sacrificing expiratory time for a longer inspiratory phase causes gas trapping and higher alveolar pressure and volumes. The commonest causes of hypotension during mechanical ventilation are dynamic hyperinflation (intrinsic or auto-positive end-expiratory pressure) sedation and pneumothorax. Hypovolaemia aggravates these causes. The treatment should be of the cause. Dynamic hyperinflation is best treated by allowing gas to empty from the lungs.

Nunn J. *Nunn's Applied Respiratory Physiology*, 4th Edn. Butterworth Heinemann, 1993.
Tuxen D in *Recent Advances* in *Critical Care Medicine 4*. Evans T, Hinds C (eds). Churchill Livingstone, 1996.

A 58. A. true   **B.** false   **C.** false   **D.** false   **E.** false

High-frequency jet ventilation (HFJV) is established in upper airway surgery but has not achieved widespread acceptance in the Intensive Care Unit despite the many potential advantages offered (lower airway pressures, improved cardiovascular stability, preservation of renal function and reduction in sedation requirements). Important variables that affect the effectiveness of HFJV are the driving pressure, ventilatory frequency and the inspiratory time, which in turn determines the I:E ratio. Adequate oxygenation and carbon dioxide removal is achieved at lower tidal volumes than those required for conventional positive pressure ventilation (1–3 ml/kg *vs* 7–10 ml/kg but they can be less than the anatomical dead space). Minute volume is dependent upon the driving pressure and I:E ratio but inversely related to the ventilatory frequency. Inadequate humidification and inadvertent alveolar gas trapping are two major potential problems when using HFJV. Humidification is technically difficult to achieve and frequently requires entrainment of gases from a second, low-pressure circuit. This method is inefficient and risks excessive patient cooling. Trapping of alveolar gas associated with this ventilatory strategy is primarily due to expiratory flow limitation. Consequently, asthma and other obstructive airway conditions are regarded as relative or absolute contraindications to the use of HFJV.

Murphy P. *Essays & MCQs in Anaesthesia and Intensive Care*. Edward Arnold, Chapter 19.

59. **A.** false **B.** true **C.** true **D.** true **E.** false

Alfentanil is shorter acting than fentanyl and does not undergo entero-systemic cycling to any clinically significant degree and has no active metabolites. This recycling phenomenon has been described with fentanyl and contributes, along with redistribution from skeletal muscle, to a risk of delayed respiratory depression. Morphine undergoes both hepatic and extrahepatic metabolism, producing both inactive (morphine-3-glucuronide) and active (morphine-6-glucuronide) metabolites with prolonged elimination half-lives. Renal failure increases the sensitivity to morphine and accumulation is therefore more likely, making the use of alfentanil in this patient group a more logical choice. With the exception of remifentanil, the first of a new generation of esterase-metabolised opioids, it should be remembered that all opioids after prolonged administration will accumulate and that clearance will then depend solely on the effectiveness of hepatorenal function. The short duration of action of midazolam in the critically ill is lost following frequent repeat dosing or prolonged infusion of the drug. This is due to the overwhelming of hepatorenal function and the accumulation of an active hydroxy-metabolite. By way of contrast, propofol has been found to be a non-cumulative sedative regardless of the mode of administration or the pre-existing state of hepatorenal function. It has been postulated that non-specific, extrahepatic esterase metabolism may contribute to the elimination of the drug, as less than 1% is excreted unchanged in the urine.

Murphy P. *Essays & MCQs in Anaesthesia and Intensive Care*. Edward Arnold, Chapter 19.

60. **A.** false **B.** true **C.** false **D.** true **E.** true

Underwater seal systems used for chest drainage are the source of much confusion and are beloved of examiners! There are three basic principles to learn. [a] The volume of the tube connecting the drain to the underwater seal must be greater than half the patient's maximal inspiratory volume to prevent water being sucked into the interpleural cavity on deep inspiration. [b] The volume of water in the underwater seal similarly needs to be greater than half the patient's maximal inspiratory volume to prevent loss of this seal and air entering the tubing on deep inspiration. [c] The depth of the tube providing the underwater seal below the surface of the water dictates the resistance to expelling air from the interpleural cavity, and hence it should be less than 5 cm. For [b] and [c] to both be true, the underwater seal bottle needs to have a broad base. A Heimlich valve is a one-way flutter valve that can be used to replace an underwater seal. In an emergency a makeshift valve can be made from the finger of a rubber glove with the end snipped off. The military have been known to use condoms in emergencies! Placed over the end of the chest drain this allows air to be expelled from a chest drain but not to enter. In situations where the drain is placed to drain both air and fluid (e.g. after cardiac surgery), then a fluid trap is utilised between the patient and the underwater seal.

Yentis, Hirsch, Smith. *Anaesthesia A to Z*. Butterworth Heinemann, 1993.

A 1.   **A.** false   **B.** false   **C.** false   **D.** false   **E.** true

A generic pacemaker code identifies pacing modes by up to five functions. Letter 1 refers to the chamber paced. Letter 2 refers to the chamber sensed. Letter 3 refers to the response to sensing (I for inhibition i.e. switched off, T for triggering). Letter 4 lists programmability (from externally): P = simple, M = complex, C = telemetry, R = adaptive. Letter 5 relates to tachyarrhythmias: P = pacing, S = DC shock, D = dual, pacing and shocks. A VVI code denotes ventricular pacing with inhibition of pacing should any spontaneous ventricular activity occur. Rate-responsive devices respond to physiological conditions that change heart rate e.g. respiration, temp, pH or haemoglobin saturation. Demand pacemakers can be converted to fixed rate by placing a magnet over them. Diathermy plates should be distant from the pacemaker and bipolar diathermy should be used if possible.

Yentis, Hirsch, Smith. *Anaesthesia A to Z.* Butterworth Heinemann.

A 2.   **A.** true   **B.** true   **C.** true   **D.** false   **E.** true

In a patient with aortic stenosis a progressive obstruction to left ventricular ejection occurs. This causes concentric left ventricular hypertrophy. The myocardium becomes susceptible to ischaemia even in the absence of coronary artery disease. In such patients the ventricle is of low compliance and atrial contraction becomes critical in maintaining ventricular filling and stroke volume. The atrial contraction accounts for up to 40% of left ventricular end-diastolic volume. Hence sinus rhythm must be ensured and atrial fibrillation cannot be ignored. Bradycardia can lead to hypotension. Slowing the heart and increasing diastolic time will not increase stroke volume; hence, bradycardia will cause a decrease in cardiac output and blood pressure. Inotropes may be helpful in the preinduction stage in severe aortic stenosis with hypotension. Ischaemia may be difficult to detect because of the electrocardiographic signs of left ventricular hypertrophy and strain.

Barash, Cullen, Stoelting. *Clinical Anesthesia*, 2nd Edn. Chapter 36.

A 3.   **A.** true   **B.** false   **C.** false   **D.** true   **E.** true

Enflurane is 2-chloro-1,1,2-trifluoroethyl difluoromethyl ether. It is a colourless volatile liquid with an ether-like odour. Its MAC value is 1.68. It does cause epileptiform EEG activity especially at high doses.

Yentis, Hirsch, Smith. *Anaesthesia A to Z*. Butterworth Heinemann, 1993.

A 4.   **A.** false   **B.** true   **C.** true   **D.** false   **E.** false

Normal cerebral blood flow is 50 ml/100 g/min and is supplied by the carotid arteries (two thirds) and the vertebral arteries (one third). The head should be maintained as near as possible to the neutral position to avoid kinking of any of these vessels perioperatively. This is particularly important but often forgotten during carotid endarterectomy. Hypoventilation results in hypercapnia which will vasodilate vessels supplying normal areas of brain, potentially leading to reduced flow to diseased areas of brain (cerebral steal syndrome). Cerebral blood flow is not increased by suxamethonium administration; however, the increase in intrathoracic pressure that occurs during fasiculation reduces cerebral venous return and thus leads to a transient rise in intracranial pressure. Cerebral blood flow is increased in a dose-dependent fashion by the administration of halothane or enflurane, although not by isoflurane at doses of up to 1 MAC.

Yentis, Hirsch, Smith. *Anaesthesia A to Z*. Butterworth Heinemann, 1993.

A 5.   **A.** false   **B.** false   **C.** true   **D.** false   **E.** false

TURP syndrome is the syndrome of intravascular volume overload and dilutional hyponatraemia related to absorption of hypotonic glycine irrigating solution through open prostatic vessels during the procedure. It presents with dyspnoea, visual and mental changes (in patients undergoing TURP under regional blockade), hyper/hypotension, angina, convulsions and coma. It may be avoided by limiting the height of the irrigant reservoir above the patient to 60 cm, limiting the length of the resection to <60 min, resection by experienced surgeons and avoidance of hypotonic IV solutions for infusion. Ethanol can be used as a marker in the irrigating fluid and can be monitored in the exhaled breath or the blood of the patient to monitor the degree of absorption.

Yentis, Hirsch, Smith. *Anaesthesia A to Z*. Butterworth Heinemann, 1993.

A 6. **A.** false   **B.** true   **C.** false   **D.** true   **E.** true

During one-lung ventilation, in the lateral position, all ventilation is directed to the lower lung but perfusion is still present in the upper lung. Hence a shunt occurs in the upper lung which may lead to hypoxaemia. In diseased lungs blood flow is usually decreased preoperatively compared to the non-diseased lung. Hence the degree of shunting is reduced in the former and the hypoxaemia is less than with one-lung ventilation in non-diseased lungs. PEEP to the ventilated lung may exacerbate hypoxaemia by reducing cardiac output or by forcing more blood to flow through the upper lung. Hypoxaemia worsens after about 10 min of one-lung ventilation as contained oxygen is absorbed. Tying the uppermost pulmonary artery stops shunting to this lung and if necessary should be performed early. Alternatively one can intermittently re-ventilate, apply CPAP or at least insufflate the upper lung with 100% oxygen.

Yentis, Hirsch, Smith. *Anaesthesia A to Z*. Butterworth Heinemann.

A 7. **A.** true   **B.** false   **C.** false   **D.** true   **E.** true

Air embolism is a potential complication of several operations but the highest risk is in spontaneously breathing neurosurgical patients who are in the sitting position for surgery. A clinically significant air embolus will cause rapid obstruction of the pulmonary vascular bed and right heart filling, causing a rise in pulmonary artery (PAP) and central venous (CVP) pressure, respectively. In most cases, the electrocardiogram will simultaneously show changes ranging from sinus tachycardia to signs of right ventricular strain and life-threatening arrhythmias. (A subsequent return of the PAP and CVP to 'pre-embolism' levels indicates successful treatment.) The classically described 'mill-wheel' murmur may be heard using an oesophageal or precordial stethoscope but is a relatively late and inconsistent sign, which may be preceded by cardiovascular collapse. In contrast, capnography provides an early and sensitive indication of air embolism before cardiovascular compromise occurs (1.5 ml air/kg). As emboli are trapped in the lung, perfusion falls causing an increase in physiological dead space. This results in a sudden fall in the peak end expired carbon dioxide concentration ($EtCO_2$). Trans-cranial doppler ultrasonography is a non-invasive method of measuring cerebral blood flow. It is a sensitive indicator of cerebrovascular spasm/embolisation but unless the patient has a patent foramen ovale (10% of adults have patent foramen ovale) it is not an appropriate means for detecting venous air emboli. Precordial (4th right intercostal space) and oesophageal doppler ultrasonography are very sensitive means of detecting systemic venous air embolism but accurate placement is essential.

Murphy P. *Essays & MCQs in Anaesthesia and Intensive Care*. Edward Arnold, Chapter 8.

A 8.   **A.** false   **B.** true   **C.** false   **D.** true   **E.** true

Preoperative arterial blood gas analysis provides a useful baseline to compare with postoperatively. Interpreted on its own, however, arterial blood oxygen tension (PaO_2) is generally considered to be a poor predictor of postoperative morbidity and mortality following lung resection for the following reasons. Firstly, PaO_2 varies with age (9 kPa is the lower limit of normal in the 70- to 79-year age group) and posture and, secondly, the portion of lung to be resected may be contributing detrimentally to a physiological shunt. Resection of lung where there is perfusion but little or no ventilation may therefore, in due course, have a beneficial effect on arterial oxygen content and subsequent exercise tolerance. In contrast, an arterial blood carbon dioxide ($PaCO_2$) tension >6 kPa has been found to correlate with an increased perioperative risk of pulmonary complications and mortality. Several studies have determined that providing the FEV_1 is >2 L (or 50% of that predicted for age, sex and height) and the FVC above 50% of its predicted value, then the patient is likely to tolerate lung resection (pneumonectomy) and no further lung function testing is required. However, if values fall significantly below these figures, particularly if FEV_1 approaches 1 L, it is advisable to undertake formal lung function testing in a pulmonary function laboratory. Some authors consider a predicted postoperative FEV_1 of 800–1,000 ml as the 'cut-off' point for pneumonectomy. (A figure calculated on the basis of functional losses, in relation to preoperative values, of 25% for lobectomy and 33% for pneumonectomy). It is now appreciated, however, that postoperative function can be more accurately determined by the state of the lung tissue to be resected. Radioisotope ventilation-perfusion scanning has been found to be a particularly useful technique for quantifying ventilation-perfusion matching prior to surgery. In patients with a marginal FEV_1, measurement of the maximum breathing capacity (MBC) may provide an additional means of identifying those patients at risk of postoperative pulmonary insufficiency. Motivation and sustainable muscle strength contribute to the successful performance of this test – factors important for a successful postoperative recovery! It is therefore not surprising that this test has been found to be reasonably predictive of subsequent morbidity and mortality.

Gothard, Kelleher. *Essentials of Cardiac and Thoracic Anaesthesia*. Butterworth Heinemann, Chapter 6.

A 9. **A.** false **B.** false **C.** false **D.** false **E.** false

Congenital pyloric stenosis usually presents in the first 2 months of life and is characterised by projectile vomiting, dehydration and electrolyte disturbances. Sodium, potassium and chloride ions are lost in the acid vomitus and the renal response to this is twofold. First, bicarbonate is excreted (combined with sodium) in an attempt to restore the pH and, secondly, potassium and hydrogen ions are excreted and sodium retained in order to minimise the reduction in extracellular volume. The first of these responses tends to produce alkaline urine and the second, an acid one. The latter, in turn, exacerbates the systemic alkalaemia resulting in further hypokalaemia. Hartmann's solution (compound sodium lactate) should be avoided in patients with metabolic alkalosis, whereas normal saline is a hydrogen ion donor and does not contribute to the bicarbonate load. This condition is a medical emergency and surgery should therefore not be contemplated until the biochemical profile has been normalised. This is achieved usually over a 24- to 48-hour period and regarded as adequately achieved when the chloride concentration is greater than

90 mmol/l, the sodium concentration is greater than 135 mmol/l and the bicarbonate concentration has fallen to less than 25 mmol/l. (An alkaline cerebrospinal fluid can result in hypoventilation and postoperative apnoea.)

Hatch, Sumner, Hellman. *The Surgical Neonate: Anaesthesia & Intensive Care*, 3rd Edn. Edward Arnold, Chapter 4.

A 10. **A.** true   **B.** true   **C.** true   **D.** false   **E.** true

Protracted nausea and vomiting (N&V) occurs in 36% of patients and is the leading cause for admission following day case surgery. Contributing factors include history of motion sickness, pain, site of surgery, opioid administration and obesity. It has been shown that laparoscopy during the menses resulted in a fourfold increase in N&V compared with at other times. Droperidol reduced the incidence with doses as low as 0.25 mg during day cases. 86% of children having strabismus surgery experienced N&V, this became 43% when given droperidol 75 μg/kg before the end of surgery. However, routine use of antiemetics in children is associated with a higher incidence of postoperative sedation and extrapyramidal side effects. The introduction of 5-HT$_3$ antagonists has helped to avoid these complications.

Barash, Cullen, Stoelting. *Clinical Anaesthesia*, 2nd Edn. Chapter 50.

A 11. **A.** true   **B.** false   **C.** true   **D.** false   **E.** true

Both soda lime and baralyme have been used for carbon dioxide absorption in anaesthetic circuits. Baralyme is no longer available in Europe but is topical because it has been cited as a potential factor in the occurrence of extreme exothermic reactions when used as a carbon dioxide absorbent in the presence of desflurane or sevoflurane (several case reports in August 2004). Soda lime consists of 94% calcium hydroxide, 5% sodium hydroxide (catalyst), and 1% potassium hydroxide and an activator. Small amounts of silica are added to produce calcium and sodium silicate, which hardens the product and reduces dust formation. Sodium hydroxide is the active carbon dioxide absorbent of soda lime. Baralyme is made of 80% calcium hydroxide and 20% barium hydroxide. Baralyme is more stable than soda lime and does not require a silica binder. Barium hydroxide is the active absorbent. Baralyme is about 15% less efficient than soda lime, by weight, at absorbing carbon dioxide. Water is required for both formulations, but baralyme already contains water, as the barium hydroxide is present as the octahydrate. Therefore, baralyme may perform better in less humid climates.

Miller. *Anesthesia*, 4th Edn. Chapter 9.

A 12. **A.** false   **B.** false   **C.** true   **D.** false   **E.** false

Most Jehovah's witnesses (JW) will not accept blood, FFP, packed cells, white cells or platelets. Cardiac bypass may be accepted as long as the pump is primed with non-blood fluids and blood is not stored in the process. Autotransfusion is acceptable to many provided the equipment is a closed circuit and constantly linked to the patient's circulation with no storage of blood. Similarly cell savers may be acceptable. Transfusion is unlawful if the patient has stipulated that they do not want to receive blood or its products. However during regional techniques and even while sedated if the need to receive blood becomes a life-saving measure then the patient may retract their prohibition under their own volition and without duress and may modify their consent if witnessed. Children over 12 years who are capable of understanding the issues may be relied upon to give consent to receive blood. Active cooling has been described in the postoperative period to decrease oxygen consumption and increase dissolved oxygen carriage but this is not widely practised.

Association of Anaesthetists of Great Britain And Ireland. *Management of Anaesthesia for Jehovah's Witnesses*. March 1999.

A 13. **A.** true   **B.** true   **C.** false   **D.** true   **E.** false

Valid consent may be given verbally as the basis of it is the explanation given to the patient. Although courts expect a greater degree of explanation than was expected in the past, a balance must be struck between telling the patient enough for informed consent to be given and not so much information as to frighten them. Consent should be obtained before the premedication is administered and the presence of a signed consent should form part of the checklist prior to departure from the ward. Written consent is not always necessary or possible e.g. the unconscious patient. In an emergency, treatment may proceed without direct patient consent if a delay would cause serious harm. A relative may not provide consent unless given prior legal guardian status by the courts, but it is preferable to try and seek it from next of kin as an exercise in diplomacy. In cases when the patient is unable to give informed consent, two consultants should document agreement that the treatment should proceed in the patient's best interests. If there is any doubt, the matter should be referred to the courts.

Association of Anaesthetists of Great Britain & Ireland. *Risk Management.* January 1998.

A 14. **A.** true **B.** true **C.** false **D.** true **E.** true

In the lateral position the lower hip and leg are at risk from pressure injury. Rhabdomyolysis can occur (more commonly in the obese) as well as arterial insufficiency and swollen thigh. A serious complication from the prone position is retinal ischaemia and blindness due to orbital compression combined with a low blood pressure. The sitting position which may still be used during neurosurgery on midline or posterior fossa structures is actually a modified recumbent position. In this position some degree of head flexion is needed. A small amount of distance must be maintained between the chin and the sternum to prevent extra- and intraoral compression ischaemia. It is known that although venous air embolism occurs more commonly in the sitting position it is not associated with any increased complication rate. Indeed there is no support for increased morbidity or mortality between the sitting position and others i.e. prone, supine or lateral. However when compared with these positions the sitting position is associated with less blood loss. The Trendelenburg position is a head down modification of the supine position and during long procedures may be associated with swollen face, eyelid, conjunctiva and tongue, so much so that lingual and buccal nerve neuropathy have occurred.

Cucchiara, Miller, Reves, Roizen, Savarese. *Anesthesia*, 4th Edn. Chapter 60.

A 15. **A.** true **B.** true **C.** true **D.** true **E.** false

The size 1 LMA can be used in newborns and patients of <5 kg, whereas the size 1.5 is appropriate for those of 5–10 kg. The size 1 has a cuff volume of up to 4 ml. The LMA provides no protection from regurgitation of stomach contents but there is evidence that it protects against contamination from oropharyngeal secretions, debris and blood. This has been demonstrated by placing methylene blue dye or barium contrast above the LMA and showing by fibreoptic studies or radiologically that none was present in the trachea. Insertion of the LMA is associated with a rise in blood pressure and heart rate of up to 20% in adults and children. They do require less depth of anaesthesia for maintenance than those who are intubated and emergence hypertension is less. Propofol used alone provides the best conditions for LMA insertion since pharyngeal and laryngeal reflexes are obtunded. Thiopentone and etomidate alone are unsuitable and may cause coughing, retching or laryngospasm. They must be combined with another drug, usually a volatile, before conditions are right. The size 5 LMA is advocated for patients weighing over 70 kg, it has an internal diameter of 11.5 mm and a cuff volume of up to 40 ml.

The Laryngeal Mask Airway. *International Anesthesiology Clinics.* Volume 36, Number 2, Lippincott-Raven, Spring 1998.

A 16. A. false **B.** false **C.** true **D.** false **E.** true

In an inguinal hernia field block, the iliohypogastric and ilioinguinal nerves are blocked by introducing a needle vertically 2 cm medial and caudal to the anterior superior iliac spine. A click is felt as the external oblique aponeurosis is penetrated. The cervical plexus is formed from the anterior branches of the upper four cervical nerves, lying between the anterior and posterior tubercles of the cervical vertebral transverse processes. They are blocked by introducing a needle 1–3 cm towards each process in turn. These are palpated posterior to a line drawn between the mastoid process and transverse process of C6. The posterior approach to blocking the sciatic nerve is performed with the patient lying with the side to be blocked uppermost with the knee flexed. A line is drawn between the greater trochanter and posterior superior iliac spine. At its midpoint a perpendicular is dropped 3 cm and the needle is introduced perpendicular to the skin. The median nerve at the wrist is blocked by passing a needle between the tendons of palmaris longus and flexor carpi radialis at the proximal palmar crease. The axillary approach to the brachial plexus is performed with the patient's head turned away, arm abducted to 90° and the hand under the head. The needle is inserted just above the axillary artery pulsation as high into the axilla as possible.

Yentis, Hirsch, Smith. *Anaesthesia A to Z*. Butterworth Heinemann.

A 17. **A.** true   **B.** true   **C.** false   **D.** false   **E.** true

Rapid IV infusion of large doses of opioids is associated with muscle rigidity. Dose and rate of administration influence this effect. The incidence can be reduced by administering the opioid over a period of >30 s. Wooden chest syndrome is a manifestation of opioid-induced muscle rigidity. It is characterised by increased muscle tone progressing to severe stiffness, particularly in the thoracic and abdominal muscles. It usually begins just after the patient loses consciousness and rarely occurs in conscious patients. A study comparing remifentanil (1 μg/kg bolus followed by 0.5 μg/kg/min) with alfentanil (25 μg/kg bolus followed by 1 μg/kg/min) showed an incidence of muscle rigidity of 8 and 5%, respectively. The actual mechanism by which opioids cause muscle rigidity is not understood. It is not due to a direct action on muscle fibres, since it can be decreased or prevented by pretreatment with muscle relaxants. Rigidity may be the result of stimulation of GABAergic interneurons. Ventilation can be impaired, but the effects can be overcome with muscle relaxation and hypnotic agents.

Thompson, Rowbotham. *BJA* 1996;76(3):341–343.
Miller. *Anesthesia*, 4th Edn.

A 18. **A.** true   **B.** false   **C.** false   **D.** true   **E.** false

Rocuronium bromide (Esmeron) is a non-depolarising muscle relaxant with an onset time that approaches that of suxamethonium. However, its duration of action is similar to that of vecuronium or atracurium. 0.6 mg/kg provides acceptable intubating conditions within 60 s. 0.45 mg/kg provides acceptable intubating conditions within 90 s. Plasma clearance is reduced in geriatric patients and those with renal impairment. In hepatic disease half-life is prolonged. Elevated plasma magnesium levels, aminoglycosides and other antibiotics may increase the effect of rocuronium while prior chronic administration of steroids, phenytoin and carbamazepine may decrease its effects. Other interactions are also described (see data sheet). It is not an MH trigger but has been implicated in a number of case reports of anaphylactic reactions.

Esmeron Data Sheet. Organon Teknika.

A **19. A.** true **B.** true **C.** false **D.** false **E.** true

This is a 'bread and butter' question which should easily allow you to pick up full marks. Sevoflurane is a methyl-propyl-ether which is unstable in soda lime. It is partly metabolised to fluoride ions. It is non-irritant. Its blood gas solubility is 0.6 and its MAC is 2%. Because it is entirely fluorinated it has a low potential to deplete the ozone layer. It is stable without additives. However, sevoflurane has been shown to produce degradation products upon interaction with carbon dioxide absorbents. The major degradation product produced is fluoromethyl-2,2-difluoro-1-(trifluoromethyl)vinyl ether, or compound A. During sevoflurane anaesthesia, factors that increase Compound A concentration include use of low-flow or closed-circuit anaesthesia, the use of baralyme rather than soda lime, higher concentrations of sevoflurane in the circuit, higher absorbent temperatures and fresh absorbent. It is said that the degradation products do not cause clinically detectable toxic effects in humans even during low-flow anaesthesia.

Aitkenhead, Smith. *Textbook of Anaesthesia*. Churchill Livingstone.
Miller. *Anesthesia*, 4th Edn. Chapter 9.

A **20. A.** true **B.** true **C.** true **D.** true **E.** true

Propofol is licensed for use as an induction agent in patients over 1 month old. Sedative infusions are not recommended for under 16 years. TCI (Target Controlled Infusion) is licensed only for adult use. Propofol protein binding is around 98%. It has little effect on bronchial muscle tone and laryngospasm is uncommon. It has antiemetic properties. Cortisol concentrations may be depressed although synacthen test should be normal.

Aitkenhead, Smith. *Textbook of Anaesthesia*. Churchill Livingstone.
BNF 38. September 1999.

A 21. **A.** true **B.** true **C.** false **D.** false **E.** false

Hydrocortisone is cortisol. 5 mg of methylprednisolone is equivalent to 4 mg of prednisolone which is equivalent to 16 mg of hydrocortisone in terms of corticosteroid activity. There is evidence that the majority of patients taking <10 mg of prednisolone long term still maintain adequate HPA activity to testing. The British Thoracic Society Guidelines on Asthma Management 1995 Review and Position Statement (BMJ Publishing Group) cites evidence that it is safe to stop a short course of steroids abruptly, clinically and in terms of plasma corticotrophin recovery. This does not mean that the disease for which the steroids were prescribed will not recur. Current recommendations err on the side of 2–3 months for safe return of HPA function.

Nicholson G et al. *Anaesthesia* 1998;53:1091–1104.

A 22. **A.** false **B.** false **C.** false **D.** true **E.** false

Barometric pressure decreases approximately exponentially with altitude. During acclimitisation, hypoxia stimulates peripheral chemoreceptors resulting in hyperventilation and respiratory alkalosis, which is corrected over the first few days by renal bicarbonate excretion. This alkalosis also results in a right shift of the oxygen dissociation curve. Although arterial PO_2 is only 45 mmHg at 15,000 ft, polycythaemia maintains oxygen delivery and the PO_2 of mixed venous blood is only a little below normal.

West. *Respiratory Physiology*, 4th Edn. Williams and Wilkins, Chapter 9.

A 23. **A.** true **B.** true **C.** false **D.** false **E.** true

Angiotensin I is formed when angiotensinogen is broken down by renin secreted from the juxta-glomerular apparatus. Prostaglandin E2 is the main one produced by the kidney and is a vasodilator. Insulin catabolism occurs in the kidney and the insulin requirements of patients with diabetes reduce as renal function decreases.

Kumar, Clark. *Clinical Medicine*, 3rd Edn. Saunders, Chapter 9.

A **24.** **A.** true **B.** true **C.** true **D.** false **E.** false

FRC is a lung capacity, the sum of residual volume and expiratory reserve volume. An average male value is 2.5–3 L. It can be measured by helium dilution, nitrogen washout or whole body plethysmography. FRC is reduced by anaesthesia, even in the presence of positive pressure ventilation. It is increased by positive end-expiratory pressure or increased airways resistance e.g. asthma.

Yentis, Hirsch, Smith. *Anaesthesia A to Z*. Butterworth Heinemann, 1993.

A **25.** **A.** true **B.** true **C.** true **D.** true **E.** true

Prys-Roberts, Brown. *International Practice of Anaesthesia*. Butterworth Heinemann, Chapter 105.

A **26.** **A.** false **B.** false **C.** true **D.** false **E.** true

Trigeminal neuralgia is characterised by attacks of 'electric-shock' like pain that usually last seconds to minutes and rarely disturb sleep. Venous or arterial involvement with the rootlets of the trigeminal nerve has been blamed for neuralgia and this may respond to surgical decompression. Two thirds of cases respond well to carbamazapine. Trigeminal neuralgia is a recognised symptom of brainstem infarction and acoustic neuromata as well as demyelinating disease.

Wall P, Melzack R. *Textbook of Pain*, 3rd Edn. Churchill Livingstone, 1994.

A **27.** **A.** true **B.** true **C.** true **D.** false **E.** true

It is estimated that more than half the UK population are infected with *Helicobacter pylori*, but only a small proportion develop peptic ulcers. Nevertheless there is strong evidence *H. pylori* is aetiological in both ulcer types, the association being stronger for duodenal ulcers. The stimulated acid secretion of parietal cells is thought to be isotonic hydrochloric acid with a pH of 0.87. The cells are protected by bicarbonate-containing mucus that maintains a surface pH of 6–7 but a gastric luminal pH of 1–2. Acute gastric mucosal injury is more frequent than duodenal but ulcers occur equally at both sites. Prospective

Exam 5

Answers

placebo-controlled trials in patients with arthritis show ranitidine is effective at preventing NSAID-induced duodenal ulcers but is ineffective against gastric ulcers. This requires omeprazole or misoprostol. Only 10–20% of peptic ulcers continue to bleed or re-bleed and so require intervention but there are high-risk groups: high volume bleeds, a haemoglobin <10 g/dl, hypotension or significant postural drop, significant co-morbidity and the elderly. In the USA patients hospitalised for NSAID-induced upper gastrointestinal bleeding have a mortality of 5–10%.

Calam J. *Medicine* 1998;26(7):11–15.
Wolfe M *et al. N Engl Med J* 1999:340:1888–1899.

A 28. A. false   **B.** true   **C.** false   **D.** false   **E.** true

The best available evidence suggests that for both primary and secondary prevention of stroke in atrial fibrillation in patients over 60, warfarin is more effective than aspirin when the international normalised ratio (INR) is greater than 2.0. Warfarin is still more effective when older than 75 but the incidence of serious haemorrhage increases and then aspirin may be of net benefit in at-risk patients. The return of muscular as opposed to electrical atrial conduction may take up to 3 weeks, and therefore anticoagulation is normally recommended to continue for at least one month. Digoxin has no place in the prevention of paroxysmal atrial fibrillation. Although digoxin may control the ventricular rate during bouts, there is evidence it prolongs attacks. Amiodarone increases plasma digoxin levels and may precipitate toxicity. Even with antiarrhythmic drug cover, >50% of patients in recent series relapse into atrial fibrillation, mostly in the first month.

Drug and Therapeutics Bulletin 1996;34(6):41–45.
Channer K. *Prescribers Journal* 1996;36(3):147–153.
Gubitz G *et al. Clinical Evidence.* BMJ Publishing Group, June 1999.

A 29. A. false   **B.** true   **C.** true   **D.** true   **E.** false

In contrast to hepatitis A, C, D and E, hepatitis B is a DNA virus. Fulminant hepatic failure occurs in less than 1%.

Kumar, Clark. *Clinical Medicine*, 3rd Edn. Saunders, Chapter 5.

A. true   **B.** false   **C.** true   **D.** true   **E.** true

Cardiac involvement in acute rheumatic fever may cause pericarditis, pericardial effusion, myocarditis or mitral valvulitis. SLE can cause pericarditis, myocarditis and non-infective endocarditis (Libman-Sachs).

Kumar, Clark. *Clinical Medicine*, 3rd Edn. Saunders, Chapter 11.

A 31. **A.** true   **B.** true   **C.** false   **D.** false   **E.** true

Apart from the obvious changes in conscious level and well-recognised increased risks of transmission of infection, the intoxicated patient may present with drug-specific problems. Cannabis produces tachycardia, abnormal affect, poor memory and fatigue. Stimulants such as cocaine, amphetamines and ecstasy (3,4-methylenedioxymethamphetamine) produce tachycardia, labile BP, excitement, delirium, hallucinations, hyper reflexia, tremors, convulsions, mydriasis, sweating, hyperpyrexia, exhaustion and coma. Hallucinogens such as LSD, phencyclidine and ketamine produce sympathomimetic effects and dissociative symptoms. Opioids are fairly predictable from the commonly observed clinical side effects. More specifically, cocaine toxicity results in intense cerbral/coronary vasospasm that can result in infarction. Additional vasopressors (even in LA solutions) may result in a hypertensive/tachydysrhythmic crisis. Ecstasy overdose commonly presents with hyperthermia (>39°C), DIC and dehydration. Excessive ADH release may also result in hyponatraemia.

Allman, Wilson. *Oxford Handbook of Anaesthesia*. OUP, 2001, Chapter 11.

A 32. **A.** false   **B.** true   **C.** false   **D.** true   **E.** true

Sarcoidosis is a non-caseating disease as opposed to some forms of tuberculosis. Sarcoid infiltration of the larynx as well as enlargement of local lymphoid tissue may increase difficulty of intubation. The associated lung disease is typically fibrotic and restrictive. Cardiac infiltration is a cause of impaired conduction, dysrhythmia and sudden complete heart block that may be aggravated by slowing of AV nodal and His-Purkinje conduction tissue by anaesthetics. Hypercalcaemia is a recognised complication. Sarcoidosis is typically steroid responsive but

Exam 5

Answers

10–20% of patients appear to have irreversible disease and 1–5% die of progressive respiratory insufficiency.

Miller RD. *Anesthesia*, 3rd Edn. 1990.
Thomas D, Mason R. *Anaesthesia* 1988;43:578–580.

A 33. **A.** true **B.** false **C.** true **D.** true **E.** true

Duchenne is the most severe and most common of the muscular dystrophies, commencing in males between 2 and 5 years of age and typically affecting proximal muscles especially the pelvis. Most are unable to walk by 10 years and die of pneumonia often by 20 years. Restrictive ventilatory defects are common from kyphoscoliosis. Cardiomyopathies are common with arrhythmias and a decreased ventricular contractility. There is no definite response to muscle relaxants but non-depolarising agents may have a prolonged recovery time and response to suxamethonium may be abnormal. There is an increased risk of malignant hyperthermia.

Nimmo, Rowbotham, Smith. *Anaesthesia*, 2nd Edn. Volume 2.

A 34. **A.** true **B.** true **C.** true **D.** true **E.** false

Even though haemorrhage may occur during delivery of the placenta, the autotransfusion of blood from the uterus may increase cardiac output by an average 80% above prepartum values. Mitral stenosis is the commonest valve lesion complicating pregnancy. Pregnancy-associated tachycardia and right ventricular stroke volume increase left atrial pressure. Pulmonary vascular disease in pregnancy both isolated or part of an Eisenmenger syndrome is associated with a high risk of death during pregnancy and a permanent deterioration in cardiac function. The modern strategy for managing warfarinised females with prosthetic heart valves is to use warfarin from conception up to a brief window of no anticoagulation for elective caesarean section and then to re-start warfarin. The overall risk of embryopathy in the first trimester is approximately 4% but the risk of valve thrombosis during heparin therapy, which may require unpredictable increases in pregnancy, is about 7%. Elective or emergency caesarean section as premature labour is common, provides a safe route for delivery for an anticoagulated neonate with minimal time without warfarin for the mother.

Oakley C. *Medicine* 1998;26(2):183–185.
Prescriber's Journal 1997;37(2).

A **35.** **A.** true **B.** false **C.** true **D.** true **E.** true

Diagnosing phaeochromocytoma involves measuring urinary vanillyl mandelic acid (a breakdown product of both noradrenaline and adrenaline), homomandellic acid (from dopamine) or direct measurements of urinary noradrenaline, adrenaline and dopamine. HIAA is measured for diagnosing carcinoid syndrome. Phaeochromocytomas are associated with multiple endocrine neoplasia Type II, and von Hippel-Lindau disease as well. Postoperative hypoglycaemia has led to serious complications in several reports. The right side may be technically more challenging in part related to the vicinity of the inferior vena cava.

Schwartz J *et al.* in *Clinical Anesthesia*, 3rd Edn. Barash P, Cullen B, Stoelting R (eds). Lippincott-Raven, 1997.
Batchelor A, Hull C. *Handbook of Clinical Anaesthesia*. Churchill Livingstone, 1996.

A **36.** **A.** true **B.** true **C.** false **D.** true **E.** false

Sulphur hexafluoride is less soluble than nitrous oxide. Nitrous oxide can therefore diffuse into an intravitreal gas bubble more rapidly than sulphur hexafluoride can diffuse out, causing a rise in intraocular pressure. Intravitreal gas may remain for up to 10 days postoperatively, so nitrous oxide should be avoided during this time. The intraocular pressure should be kept normal for scleral banding, or the band will become too loose or too tight following anaesthesia.

Prys-Roberts, Brown. *International Practice of Anaesthesia*. 1st Edn. Butterworth Heinemann, Chapter 110.

A **37.** **A.** true **B.** false **C.** false **D.** true **E.** true

Thyroid storm may occur in patients during or after thyroid surgery. It presents as rapidly increasing temperature, tachycardia and hypermetabolism. Hypoparathyroidism may occur after surgery. Patients who are thyrotoxic should be made euthyroid preoperatively using antithyroid drugs (e.g. propylthiouracil).

Prys-Roberts, Brown. *International Practice of Anaesthesia.* Butterworth Heinemann, Chapter 82.

A 38. A. true **B.** false **C.** false **D.** false **E.** false

Complications of infection, fluid and electrolyte balance and hypothermia mandate early surgery for neonates with gastroschisis. Intact peritoneum around an exomphalocele may allow repair to be delayed. Exomphalos is associated with many other abnormalities such as Beckwith-Wiedemann syndrome and the Pentalogy of Cantrell. Gastroschisis is usually a unique abnormality as it may be caused by intrauterine occlusion of the omphalomesenteric artery. Primary closure may be impossible due to intrabdominal pressure impairing venous return, visceral perfusion and ventilation. Most neonates require a few days of mechanical ventilation. Mode of delivery is usually by caesarean section when planned but advocates of vaginal delivery point out that most infants with these defects are born vaginally without bowel injury.

Berry F in Clinical Anaesthesia, 3rd Edn. Barash P, Cullen B, Stoelting R (eds). Lippincott-Raven, 1997.

A 39. A. true **B.** true **C.** false **D.** false **E.** false

Electrolytic solutions such as Hartmann's and normal saline do least harm when absorbed into the circulation but inhibit the cutting properties of the resectoscope by dispersing its cutting current. TURP syndrome is caused by an increase in circulating blood volume and dilution of serum electrolytes. It is manifested by increased systolic, diastolic and pulse pressure. In an awake patient restlessness, nausea, vomiting, mental confusion, muscle twitching and visual disturbances may occur. These symptoms may progress to hypotension, arrhythmias, cyanosis, dyspnoea and fits. The ideal irrigant should be non-ionic, non-toxic and non-haemolytic. Glycine and Cytal (sorbitol 2.7% and mannitol 0.54%) are commonly used. They are non-haemolytic. Elderly patients have reduced autonomic nervous system function leading to thermoregulatory impairment. Hypothermia itself may cause confusion during anaesthesia. It is not influenced by anaesthetic choice. General anaesthesia decreases overall heat production, whereas regionals have no effect on it. However, after the end of a general anaesthetic, oxygen uptake and plasma catecholamines are increased, whereas no such changes occur after regional anaesthetic. The incidence of bladder perforation is 0.9–1.1% and most are extraperitoneal. They cause abdominal pain in the conscious patient with diaphragmatic irritation if intraperitoneal. Small perforations may be managed conservatively with catheter drainage.

Barash, Cullen, Stoelting. *Clinical Anesthesia*, 2nd Edn. Chapter 41.

A 40. A. true **B.** true **C.** true **D.** true **E.** true

Normal portal pressure is 5–10 mmHg. If vasopressin is used, GTN may be added to reduce cardiovascular side effects.

McLatchie. *Oxford Handbook of Clinical Surgery*, 1st Edn. Oxford Medical Publications, Chapter 5.

A 41. A. true **B.** true **C.** false **D.** false **E.** false

CVP catheter monitoring actually measures mean intrathoracic pressure. Hence, in the presence of low chest wall/lung compliance, the CVP in a spontaneously ventilating patient may be underestimated, and in a mechanically ventilated patient may be overestimated. The 'a' wave in the CVP trace results from atrial contraction, hence it disappears in the presence of atrial fibrillation. Third degree heart block causes the right atrium to contract against a closed tricuspid valve, causing cannon waves. Tricuspid regurgitation produces giant 'v' waves.

Nimmo, Rowbotham, Smith. *Anaesthesia*, 2nd Edn. Blackwell Scientific Publications, Chapter 35.

A 42. A. false **B.** true **C.** false **D.** true **E.** true

Oxygen is paramagnetic and is, therefore, attracted to a magnetic field. Most other gases are weakly diamagnetic and are repelled from a magnetic field. The paramagnetic property of oxygen is due to the presence of unpaired electrons in the outer shell of the molecule. The paramagnetic analyser is a gas-tight chamber with two nitrogen-filled spheres and a rotating dumb bell in a non-uniform magnetic field. Oxygen displaces the spheres and the dumb bell rotates. Displacement may be measured by the reflection of a light beam on to a mirror. Alternatively, in the null deflection technique the light beam falls onto photocells and another current is generated to produce an opposing magnetic field. These are very accurate (around 0.1%). Calibration is required. The fuel call has a gold cathode and lead anode. The cell produces a voltage, acting as its own battery. The quadripole mass spectrometer channels a gas sample through an ionisation chamber and focusing electrode. Ions then pass through the quadripole. Rapid changes in the applied electric fields cause all ions except those with the chosen charge:mass ratio to hit the sides of the instrument. The ions of interest are registered when they strike the target at the other end.

Parbrook GD, Davis PD, Parbrook EO. *Basic Physics and Measurement in anaesthesia*. Butterworth Heinnemann.

A 43. A. true **B.** true **C.** false **D.** false **E.** false

SI units were introduced in 1960 by the General Conference of Weights and Measures; based on the metric system there are seven base units (metre, second, kilogram, ampere, kelvin, candela and mole). The following are, strictly speaking, derived units (Newton, Pascal, Watt, Joule and Hertz.)

Yentis, Hirsch, Smith. *Anaesthesia A to Z*. Butterworth Heinemann.

A 44. A. false **B.** true **C.** true **D.** true **E.** false

The TEC 6 vaporiser is specifically designed to deliver desflurane. To overcome the difficulties of a high MAC (6%), unpredictable vaporisation at 20°C, and an SVP that is close to atmospheric pressure (desflurane has a boiling point of 23.5°C and an SVP of 664 mmHg), the vaporiser is electrically heated to maintain a constant 39°C in the vaporisation sump. Here ambient pressure is maintained at 2 atmospheres. An independent fresh gas flow is mixed downstream and pressure is autoregulated to maintain a pressure of 1.1 atmospheres at a fresh gas flow of 10 L/min. Therefore, unlike contemporary variable-bypass vaporisers, the Tec 6 vaporiser requires manual adjustments of the concentration control dial at altitudes other than sea level to maintain a constant partial pressure of anaesthetic. Since it is working at its own pressure, altitude does not affect its output, and it will accurately deliver the dialled volumes percent of desflurane but this does not equal an accurate partial pressure of anaesthetic. To compensate for the reduction in partial pressure, the set concentration on the dial must be increased to maintain the required anaesthetic partial pressure. For example, at an altitude of 2,000 m, the anaesthetist would have to manually increase the concentration control dial from 10–12.8% to maintain the required anaesthetic partial pressure.

Miller. *Anesthesia*, 4th Edn. Chapters 9 and 71.

A **45. A.** true **B.** false **C.** false **D.** true **E.** false

The pneumotachograph provides a continuous measurement of airflow. It measures the drop in pressure across a gauze screen, which is then transduced into an electrical signal. Because the screen is large, flow remains laminar. The pneumotachograph can measure rapid changes in respiration with the advantage of imposing minimal resistance. However, temperature changes may affect the calibration of the pneumotachograph. The bubble flowmeter has a fixed orifice and the system is not dependent on the composition of the gases flowing.

Parbrook GD, Davis PD, Parbrook EO. *Basic Physics and Measurement in Anaesthesia*. Butterworth Heinnemann.

A **46. A.** false **B.** true **C.** false **D.** true **E.** false

The oxygen electrode consists of a silver/silver chloride anode and platinum cathode. The electrolyte solution is commonly potassium chloride. Electrons are provided at the anode by the reaction of silver with the chloride ions of the electrolyte solution. At the cathode oxygen combines with electrons and water to produce hydroxyl ions. The more oxygen available, the greater the current flow. The cathode cannot be inserted directly into blood because of protein deposition. To overcome this a plastic membrane can be used to separate electrolyte from blood.

Parbrook GD, Davis PD, Parbrook EO. *Basic Physics and Measurement in Anaesthesia*. Butterworth Heinnemann.

A **47.** **A.** false   **B.** true   **C.** false   **D.** true   **E.** false

Indications for thrombolytic therapy include presentation within 12 h with chest pain suggestive of an MI and: ST segment elevation >0.2 mV in 2 adjacent chest leads, or >0.1 mV in 2 or more limb leads; or dominant R waves and ST depression in V1–3 (posterior MI) or new-onset LBBB. Presentation 12–24 h after onset with continuing pain +/− ECG evidence of an evolving infarct is also an indication. Absolute contraindications to thrombolysis include: previous haemorrhagic stroke, CVA within 6 months, active internal bleeding (menses excluded) and aortic dissection. Streptokinase is given as 1.5 million units in 100 ml saline over 1 h. Alteplase is given as 15 mg IV bolus followed by 0.75 mg/kg over 1 h then 48 h of heparin therapy. Reteplase is given as 10 units IV bolus followed by 10 units IV bolus after 30 min then 48 h of heparin therapy.

Resuscitation Council (UK). *Advanced Life Support Provider Manual*, ISBN 1–903812–05–4.

A **48.** **A.** true   **B.** false   **C.** false   **D.** true   **E.** true

Although both nitric oxide and ECMO are used in the treatment of ARDS, neither has been shown to improve outcome and consequently they should still be considered experimental techniques rather than accepted treatment strategies. Corticosteroids have been shown to be beneficial during the fibrosing stage of ARDS but this benefit seems to be limited to a narrow therapeutic window (between 7 and 15 days after the onset of ARDS).

Oh. T *Intensive Care Manual*, 4th Edn. Butterworth Heinemann, Chapter 29. Craft TM, Nolan JP, Parr MJA. *Key Topics in Critical Care, 1st Edn*. BIOS Scientific Publishers Ltd.

A **49.** **A.** false   **B.** true   **C.** false   **D.** false   **E.** false

Calcium replacement should be titrated against ionised calcium, not total serum calcium. Although hard evidence regarding when and how to feed is lacking, current consensus recommends that nasojejunal feeding should be initiated and only if this is not tolerated should it be replaced with parenteral nutrition. Thoracic epidural is the analgesic method of choice if there are no contraindications. Where systemic opioids are required morphine is still probably a better choice of drug than pethidine in spite of theoretical concerns that it causes spasm of the sphincter of Oddi. Drainage of a pancreatic pseudocyst should be considered if the pseudocyst is greater than 5–6 cm in diameter, causing gastric outlet obstruction, if there is infection or haemorrhage into the cyst, or if it is causing pain.

Craft TM, Nolan JP, Parr MJA. *Key Topics in Critical Care*, 1st Edn. BIOS Scientific Publishers Ltd.

A **50.** **A.** false   **B.** true   **C.** true   **D.** false   **E.** true

Normal values for PA catheter measurements include:
$CI = 2.5–4.0\,L/min/m^2$
$SVR = 1{,}200–1{,}500\ dynes \cdot cm \cdot s^{-5}$
$PVR = 100–300\ dynes \cdot cm \cdot s^{-5}$
Septic shock is a hyperdynamic state and therefore presents with a raised cardiac output, unless there is a mixed picture due to co-existent myocardial disease. A raised pulmonary capillary wedge pressure suggests myocardial dysfunction rather than septic shock.

Oh T. *Intensive Care Manual*, 4th Edn. Butterworth Heinemann. Chapter 61.

A **51.** **A.** true   **B.** false   **C.** false   **D.** false   **E.** false

The ever popular anion gap crops up frequently in MCQs and is defined as $= [K^+] + [Na^+] - [Cl^-] - [HCO_3^-]$ plasma concentrations. It is a measure of the difference between unmeasured anions and cations and has a 'normal' value of 8–16 mmol/L. This question is complicated by the need to establish two truths within each leaf. This basic requirement is often overlooked if each leaf is not read in conjunction with the question stem.
Metabolic acidosis (raised AG): acid ingestion (not Cl^- ions); acid from metabolism; trauma.
Metabolic acidosis (normal AG): failure to excrete acid; renal disease; loss of base; accumulation of HCl^-.
Metabolic alkalosis: loss of H^+ ions, ingestion of base; vomiting; burns; hypokalaemia.

Oh T. *Intensive Care Manual*, 4th Edn. Butterworth Heinemann, Chapter 80.

A 52. **A.** true **B.** false **C.** true **D.** false **E.** false

The most important factor in a good outcome following drowning is early on-scene basic life support. Defibrillation is unlikely to be successful until the patient has been warmed to a core temperature of 30°C and drugs should be withheld or dose-adjusted until this point because of the risk of accumulation with decreased metabolism at low body temperatures. When immersed in cold water in outdoor clothing, core temperature falls slowly. When core temperature falls to 33–35°C, muscles are generally much colder, resulting in poor neuromuscular performance and a high risk of aspiration. This occurs long before any temperature-related neuroprotection. There is no evidence that steroids improve outcome.

Oh T. *Intensive Care Manual*, 4th Edn. Butterworth Heinemann, 1997.
Craft TM, Nolan JP, Parr MJA. *Key Topics in Intensive Care*. 1st Edn. BIOS Scientific Publishers.

A 53. **A.** true **B.** true **C.** true **D.** true **E.** true

Although not routinely used, nitroglycerin, calcium-channel blockers, inhaled clonidine and IV glucagon have all been shown to improve bronchospasm. Magnesium is now recommended by the British Thoracic Society for use in severe refractory asthma or life-threatening asthma (up to 2 g IV). Aminophylline, in addition to its bronchodilating properties, increases cardiac output and diaphragmatic contractility and may have an anti-inflammatory effect. Toxic effects, however, limit its use. Treatment with β-agonists can cause a transient increase in V/Q mismatch but supplementary oxygen alleviates this problem.

Oh T. *Intensive Care Manual*. 4th Edn. Butterworth Heinemann, 1997.
Drugs & Therapeutics Bulletin, Volume 41, Number 10, October 2003.

A 54. **A.** true **B.** false **C.** true **D.** true **E.** true

There are numerous risk factors for pulmonary embolism. These are some of the less common ones. Polycythaemia rather than anaemia is a risk factor.

Oh T. *Intensive Care Manual*, 4th Edn. Butterworth Heinemann, 1997, Chapter 30.

A 55. A. false **B.** true **C.** true **D.** false **E.** false

Parenteral nutrition carries a risk of infection but this must be balanced against the negative aspects of failure to provide nutrition if the enteral route is not available. Aseptic precautions should be observed in all cases, with particular attention paid to central line access. Infected lines should be removed or replaced. Nutritional support of septic patients is designed to reduce glucose administration because plasma glucose levels are frequently high and peripheral tissues cannot use it as a substrate. Lipid emulsions are used because fatty acids and ketone bodies are the preferred calorie source for many organs during sepsis. Amino acid mixtures are enriched with branched-chain amino acids to provide another non-glucose fuel source for skeletal muscle and to prevent muscle breakdown. The feeds are hyperosmolar and irritant to veins.

Miller RD. *Anesthesia*, 4th Edn. Chapter 78.

A 56. A. true **B.** true **C.** true **D.** true **E.** true

Propofol can cause greenish urine. Rifampicin causes all body secretions to turn red. Beetroot also causes dark-coloured urine. Patients taking L-dopa and those with porphyria may develop discoloured urine after it has been standing for some time.

Kumar, Clark. *Clinical Medicine*, 3rd Edn. Saunders, Chapter 9.

A 57. A. true **B.** true **C.** false **D.** true **E.** false

X-ray contrast medium (e.g. 'Omnipaque' - a non-ionic, monomeric, triiodinated water-soluble compound) is used in both adults and children for urography, phlebography, CT, angiography, myelography, arthrography, ERP/ERCP, hysterosalpingography, sialography and other investigations. The quoted brand is isotonic with blood at its weakest solution of 140 mg/ml but is more often used in its 300 mg/ml form. Its use is contraindicated in the presence of thyrotoxicosis (because of the effect of the iodide load) and in patients who have suffered previous reactions to it. Special caution should be exercised with patients who have a positive history of asthma, allergy or previous reactions to iodinated contrast media. Anaphylactoid reaction is more likely than anaphylaxis. Infants and neonates are susceptible to electrolyte and haemodynamic disturbance. Pulmonary hypertension and serious cardiac disease predisposes the patient to dysrhythmias. Those with cerebral pathology, epilepsy, alcoholics and drug addicts have an increased risk of experiencing seizures. Myelography can result in temporary or even permanent deafness, but this may be due to a subsequent drop in CSF pressure. Patients with diabetes, paraproteinaemia or renal impairment are at risk of developing acute renal failure. Patients already on haemodialysis can be given contrast provided dialysis is performed immediately afterwards. Iodinated contrast aggravates myasthenia gravis, phaeochromocytoma (hypertension unless α-blocked) and hyperthyroidism (can turn a multinodular thyroid hyperthyroid due to iodide uptake). The contrast may interact with biguanides (lactic acidosis), thyroid function tests, and serum bilirubin, calcium, iron and phosphate assays. So these should not be performed until the day following the investigation.

'Omnipaque' (Iohexol) Data Sheet. Nycomed, January 1999.

A 58. A. false **B.** true **C.** false **D.** true **E.** true

Ranson's criteria form the most popular scoring system to assess the severity of pancreatitis. They comprise 5 criteria assessed on admission (age over 55 years, WBC over 16,000/mm^3, glucose over 11 mmol/L, LDH over 350 IU/L, AST over 250 U/L) and 6 criteria assessed at 48 h (reduction in haematocrit of at least 10%, increase in blood urea of greater than 1.8 mmol/L, serum calcium below 2 mmol/L, PaO$_2$ less than 8 kPa, base deficit greater than 4 mmol/L, fluid sequestration greater than 6 L). The presence of less than 3 criteria is associated with a mortality below 1%, 3–4 criteria with a mortality of 16% and 5 or more is associated with a mortality of greater than 40%. The Imrie score reduces the number of Ranson's criteria by 3 (LDH, base deficit and fluid sequestration) without losing predictive power.

Craft TM, Nolan JP, Parr MJA. *Key Topics in Critical Care.* BIOS Scientific Publishers.

A 59. A. true **B.** true **C.** false **D.** true **E.** false

Acute coronary syndromes include: unstable angina, non-Q wave myocardial infarction and Q wave infarction. Fissuring of an atheromatous plaque in the wall of a coronary artery triggers haemorrhage into the plaque, arterial wall smooth muscle contraction, and thrombus formation within the vessel lumen. All these contribute to a reduction in blood flow through the affected coronary artery. Unstable angina differs from stable angina of effort, which ceases promptly on cessation of exercise. Stable angina that becomes more frequent over a few days and is related to less and less effort is regarded as unstable and is termed crescendo angina. Adverse prognostic signs on a presenting ECG include ST depression, evidence of infarction and the presence of new left bundle branch block. Reperfusion therapy should be considered in all patients with an acute MI accompanied by ST elevation or new left bundle branch block. Most patients with cardiac ischaemic pain are more comfortable sitting up.

Resuscitation Council (UK). *Advanced Life Support Provider Manual*, ISBN 1–903812–05–4.

A 60. **A.** false   **B.** true   **C.** false   **D.** true   **E.** true

The Q-T interval is measured from the first deflection of the QRS complex to the end of the T wave. It is corrected for different rates by dividing the Q-T interval by the square root of the cycle length. Changes in the length of the Q-T interval may therefore be physiological (lengthens with decreasing heart rate) or pathological in origin. Hypocalcaemia, hypothermia, ischaemic heart disease and myocarditis are all acquired causes of a prolonged Q-T interval. Jervell-Lange-Nielsen and Romano-Ward syndromes are rare congenital causes of Q-T prolongation which should be considered in patients with unexplained Q-T prolongation on their preoperative ECG and a strong family history of sudden death. Pericarditis may complicate a recent myocardial infarction but unless associated with an underlying myocarditis is typified on the 12-lead ECG by symmetrical S-T elevation (concave upwards) in all leads with the exception of aVR, where there is often S-T depression. Hyperparathyroidism results in hypercalcaemia.

Murphy P. *Essays & MCQs in Anaesthesia & Intensive Care*. Edward Arnold, Chapter 4.
Kumar, Clark. *Clinical Medicine*, 2nd Edn. Bailliere Tindall, Chapter 11.

NOTES

NOTES

NOTES

NOTES

NOTES